HANDBOOK

Fourth Edition
February 2001

Lead Editor:
LTC Mark Kortepeter

Contributing Editors:
LTC George Christopher
COL Ted Cieslak
CDR Randall Culpepper
CDR Robert Darling
MAJ Julie Pavlin
LTC John Rowe
LTC Scott Stanek

Senior Editors:
COL Edward Eitzen, Jr.
COL Kelly McKee, Jr.

Comments and suggestions are appreciated and should be addressed to:

Operational Medicine Division
Attn: MCMR-UIM-O
U.S. Army Medical Research
Institute of Infectious Diseases (USAMRIID)
Fort Detrick, Maryland 21702-5011

PREFACE TO THE FOURTH EDITION

The Medical Management of Biological Casualties Handbook, which has become affectionately known as the "Blue Book," has been enormously successful - far beyond our expectations. Since the first edition in 1993, the awareness of biological weapons in the United States has increased dramatically. Over 100,000 copies have been distributed to military and civilian health care providers around the world, primarily through USAMRIID's on-site and road Medical Management of Biological Casualties course and its four annual satellite broadcasts on this subject.

This fourth edition has been completely re-edited and updated. New chapters have been added on melioidosis, the medical management of a biological weapon attack, and the use of epidemiologic clues in determining whether an outbreak might have been intentionally spread. In addition, a reference appendix has been added for those interested in more in-depth reading on this subject.

Our goal is to make this a reference for the health care provider on the front lines, whether on the battlefield or in a clinic, who needs basic summary and treatment information quickly. We believe we have been successful in this regard. We appreciate any feedback that might make future editions more useful. Thank you for your interest in this important subject.

ACKNOWLEDGMENTS

This handbook would not be possible without the generous assistance and support of LTC(P) Les Caudle (editor of prior editions), Dr. Richard Dukes, COL(ret) David Franz, COL Gerald Parker, COL Gerald Jennings, SGM Raymond Alston, COL James Arthur, COL W. Russell Byrne, Dr. John Ezzell, COL Arthur Friedlander, Dr. Robert Hawley, COL Erik Henchal, COL(ret) Ted Hussey, Dr. Peter Jahrling, LTC Ross LeClaire, Dr. George Ludwig, Mr. William Patrick, Dr. Mark Poli, Dr. Fred Sidell, Dr. Jonathon Smith, Mr. Richard Stevens, Dr. Jeff Teska, COL Stanley Wiener and others too numerous to mention. The exclusion of anyone on this page is purely accidental and in no way lessens the gratitude we feel for contributions received.

DISCLAIMER

The purpose of this Handbook is to provide concise supplemental reading material to assist in education of biological casualty management. Although every effort has been made to make the information in this handbook consistent with official policy and doctrine (see FM 8-284), the information contained in this handbook is **not** official Department of the Army policy or doctrine, and it should not be construed as such.

As you review this handbook, you will find specific therapies and prophylactic regimens for the diseases mentioned. The majority of these are based on standard treatment guidelines; however some of the regimens noted may vary from information found in standard reference materials. The reason for this is that the clinical presentation of certain biological weapon diseases may vary from the endemic form of the disease. For ethical reasons, human challenge studies can only be done with a limited number of these agents. Therefore, treatment and prophylaxis regimens may be derived from in vitro data, animal models, and limited human data. Occasionally you will find various investigational new drug (IND) products mentioned. They are often used in the laboratory setting to protect healthcare workers. These products are not available commercially, and can only be given under a specific protocol with informed consent. They are mentioned for scientific completeness of the handbook, and are not necessarily to be construed as recommendations for therapy.

EXECUTIVE ORDER 13139:
IMPROVING HEALTH PROTECTION OF MILITARY PERSONNEL PARTICIPATING IN PARTICULAR MILITARY OPERATIONS

On 30 September 1999, the President of the United States issued Executive Order 13139, which outlines the conditions under which IND and off-label pharmaceuticals could be administered to U.S. service members. This handbook discusses numerous pharmaceutical products, some of which are investigational new drugs (IND). In certain other cases, licensed pharmaceuticals are discussed for use in a manner or for a condition other than that for which they were originally licensed (i.e. An "off-label" indication).

This executive order does not intend to alter the traditional physician-patient relationship or individual physician prescribing practices. Health care providers remain free to exercise clinical judgement and prescribe licensed pharmaceutical products as they deem appropriate for the optimal care of their patients. This policy does, however, potentially influence recommendations that might be made by U.S. government agencies and that might be applied to large numbers of service members outside of the individual physician-patient relationship. The following text presents a brief overview of EO 13139 for the benefit of the individual provider.

EO13139:

- Provides the Secretary of Defense guidance regarding the provision of IND products or products unapproved for their intended use as antidotes to chemical, biological, or radiological weapons;

- Stipulates that the US Government will administer products approved by the Food and Drug Administration (FDA) only for their intended use;

- Provides the circumstances and controls under which IND products may be used.

In order to administer an IND product:

- Informed consent must be obtained from individual service members;

- The President may waive informed consent (at the request of the Secretary of Defense and only the Secretary of Defense) if:
  - Informed consent is not feasible
  - Informed consent is contrary to the best interests of the service member
  - Obtaining informed consent is not in the best interests of national security.

Introduction

Bacterial Agents

Viral Agents

Biological Toxins

Detection

Personal Protection

Decontamination

Appendix A-K

Table of Contents

Introduction	1
History of Biological Warfare and Current Threat	3
Distinguishing Between Natural and Intentional Disease Outbreaks	11
Ten Steps in the Management of Biological Casualties on the Battlefield	15
Bacterial Agents	24
Anthrax	26
Brucellosis	36
Glanders and Melioidosis	44
Plague	53
Q Fever	62
Tularemia	69
Viral Agents	78
Smallpox	79
Venezuelan Equine Encephalitis	89
Viral Hemorrhagic Fevers	99
Biological Toxins	116
Botulinum	118
Ricin	130
Staphylococcal Enterotoxin B	138
T-2 Mycotoxins	146
Detection	154
Personal Protection	156
Decontamination	161

Appendix A: Glossary of Medical Terms
Appendix B: Patient Isolation Precautions
Appendix C: BW Agent Characteristics

Appendix D: BW Agent Vaccines, Therapeutics and Prophylactics

Appendix E: Medical Sample Collection for BW Agents

Appendix F: Specimens for Laboratory Diagnosis

Appendix G: BW Agent Laboratory Identification

Appendix H: Differential Diagnosis - Toxins vs. Nerve Agents

Appendix I: Comparative Lethality - Toxins vs. Chemical Agents

Appendix J: Aerosol Toxicity

Appendix K: References and Emergency Response Contacts

INTRODUCTION

Medical defense against biological warfare or terrorism is an area of study unfamiliar to most military and civilian health care providers during peacetime. In the aftermath of Operations Desert Shield/Desert Storm, it became obvious that the threat of biological attacks against our soldiers was real. Increased incidents and threats of domestic terrorism (e.g., New York City World Trade Center bombing, Tokyo subway sarin release, Oklahoma City federal building bombing, Atlanta Centennial Park bombing) as well as numerous anthrax hoaxes around the country have brought the issue home to civilians as well. Other issues, including the disclosure of a sophisticated offensive biological warfare program in the Former Soviet Union (FSU), have reinforced the need for increased training and education of health care professionals on how to prevent and treat biological warfare casualties.

Numerous measures to improve preparedness for and response to biological warfare or terrorism are ongoing at local, state, and federal levels. Training efforts have increased both in the military and civilian sectors. The Medical Management of Chemical and Biological Casualties Course taught at both USAMRIID and USAMRICD trains over 560 military medical professionals each year on both biological and chemical medical defense. The highly successful 3-day USAMRIID satellite course on the Medical Management of Biological Casualties has reached over 40,000 medical personnel over the last three years.

Through this handbook and the training courses noted above, medical professionals will learn that effective medical countermeasures are available against many of the bacteria, viruses, and toxins which might be used as biological weapons against our military forces or civilian communities. The importance of this education cannot be overemphasized and it is hoped that our physicians, nurses, and allied medical professionals will develop a solid understanding of the biological threats we face and the medical armamentarium useful in defending against these threats.

The global biological warfare threat is serious, and the potential for devastating casualties is high for certain biological agents. There are at least 10 countries around the world currently that have offensive biological weapons programs. However, with appropriate use of medical countermeasures either already developed or under development, many casualties can be prevented or minimized.

The purpose for this handbook is to serve as a concise pocket-sized manual that will guide medical personnel in the prophylaxis and management of biological casualties. It is designed as a quick reference and overview, and is not intended as a definitive text on the medical management of biological casualties.

HISTORY OF BIOLOGICAL WARFARE AND CURRENT THREAT

The use of biological weapons in warfare has been recorded throughout history. Two of the earliest reported uses occurred in the 6th century BC, with the Assyrians poisoning enemy wells with rye ergot, and Solon's use of the purgative herb hellebore during the siege of Krissa. In 1346, plague broke out in the Tartar army during its siege of Kaffa (at present day Feodosia in Crimea). The attackers hurled the corpses of plague victims over the city walls; the plague epidemic that followed forced the defenders to surrender, and some infected people who left Kaffa may have started the Black Death pandemic which spread throughout Europe. Russian troops may have used the same tactic against Sweden in 1710.

On several occasions, smallpox was used as a biological weapon. Pizarro is said to have presented South American natives with variola-contaminated clothing in the 15th century, and the English did the same when Sir Jeffery Amherst provided Indians loyal to the French with smallpox-laden blankets during the French and Indian War of 1754 to 1767. Native Americans defending Fort Carillon sustained epidemic casualties which directly contributed to the loss of the fort to the English.

In this century, there is evidence that during World War I, German agents inoculated horses and cattle with glanders in the U.S. before the animals were shipped to France. In 1937, Japan started an ambitious biological warfare program, located 40 miles south of Harbin, Manchuria, in a laboratory complex code-named "Unit 731". Studies directed by Japanese General Ishii continued there until 1945, when the complex was burned. A post World War II investigation revealed that the Japanese researched numerous organisms and used prisoners of war as research subjects. Slightly less than 1,000 human autopsies apparently were carried out at Unit 731, mostly on victims exposed to aerosolized anthrax. Many more prisoners and Chinese nationals may have died in this facility - some have estimated up to 3,000 human deaths. Following reported overflights by Japanese planes suspected of dropping plague-infected fleas, a plague epidemic ensued in China and Manchuria. By 1945, the Japanese program had stockpiled 400 kilograms of anthrax to be used in a specially designed fragmentation bomb.

In 1943, the United States began research into the use of biological agents for offensive purposes. This work was started, interestingly enough, in response to a perceived German biological warfare (BW) threat as opposed to a Japanese one. The United States conducted this research at Camp Detrick (now Fort Detrick), which was a small National Guard airfield prior to that time, and produced agents at other sites until 1969, when President Nixon stopped all offensive biological and toxin weapon research and production by executive order. Between May 1971 and May 1972, all stockpiles of biological agents and munitions from the now defunct U.S. program were destroyed in the presence of monitors representing the United States

Department of Agriculture, the Department of Health, Education, and Welfare, and the states of Arkansas, Colorado, and Maryland. Included among the destroyed agents were *Bacillus anthracis*, botulinum toxin, *Francisella tularensis*, *Coxiella burnetii*, Venezuelan equine encephalitis virus, *Brucella suis*, and Staphylococcal enterotoxin B. The United States began a medical defensive program in 1953 that continues today at USAMRIID.

In 1972, the United States, UK, and USSR signed the Convention on the Prohibition of the Development, Production and Stockpiling of Bacteriological (Biological) and Toxin Weapons and on Their Destruction, commonly called the Biological Weapons Convention. Over 140 countries have since added their ratification. This treaty prohibits the stockpiling of biological agents for offensive military purposes, and also forbids research into such offensive employment of biological agents. However, despite this historic agreement among nations, biological warfare research continued to flourish in many countries hostile to the United States. Moreover, there have been several cases of suspected or actual use of biological weapons. Among the most notorious of these were the "yellow rain" incidents in Southeast Asia, the use of ricin as an assassination weapon in London in 1978, and the accidental release of anthrax spores at Sverdlovsk in 1979.

Testimony from the late 1970's indicated that Laos and Kampuchea were attacked by planes and helicopters delivering aerosols of several colors. After being exposed, people and animals became disoriented and ill, and a small percentage of those stricken died. Some of these clouds were thought to be comprised of trichothecene toxins (in particular, T2 mycotoxin). These attacks are grouped under the label "yellow rain". There has been a great deal of controversy about whether these clouds were truly biological warfare agents. Some have argued that the clouds were nothing more than feces produced by swarms of bees.

In 1978, a Bulgarian exile named Georgi Markov was attacked in London with a device disguised as an umbrella. The device injected a tiny pellet filled with ricin toxin into the subcutaneous tissue of his leg while he was waiting for a bus. He died several days later. On autopsy, the tiny pellet was found and determined to contain the toxin. It was later revealed that the Bulgarian secret service carried out the assassination, and the technology to commit the crime was supplied by the former Soviet Union.

In April, 1979, an incident occurred in Sverdlovsk (now Yekaterinburg) in the former Soviet Union which appeared to be an accidental aerosol release of *Bacillus anthracis* spores from a Soviet Military microbiology facility: Compound 19. Residents living downwind from this compound developed high fever and difficulty breathing, and a large number died. The Soviet Ministry of Health blamed the deaths on the consumption of contaminated meat, and for years controversy raged in the press over the actual cause of the outbreak. All evidence available to the United States government indicated a massive release of aerosolized

B. anthracis spores. In the summer of 1992, U.S. intelligence officials were proven correct when the new Russian President, Boris Yeltsin, acknowledged that the Sverdlovsk incident was in fact related to military developments at the microbiology facility. In 1994, Meselson and colleagues published an in-depth analysis of the Sverdlovsk incident (*Science* 266:1202-1208). They documented that all of the cases from 1979 occurred within a narrow zone extending 4 kilometers downwind in a southerly direction from Compound 19. There were 66 fatalities of the 77 patients identified.

In August, 1991, the United Nations carried out its first inspection of Iraq's biological warfare capabilities in the aftermath of the Gulf War. On August 2, 1991, representatives of the Iraqi government announced to leaders of United Nations Special Commission Team 7 that they had conducted research into the offensive use of *Bacillus anthracis*, botulinum toxins, and *Clostridium perfringens* (presumably one of its toxins). This open admission of biological weapons research verified many of the concerns of the U.S. intelligence community. Iraq had extensive and redundant research facilities at Salman Pak and other sites, many of which were destroyed during the war.

In 1995, further information on Iraq's offensive program was made available to United Nations inspectors. Iraq conducted research and development work on anthrax, botulinum toxins, *Clostridium perfringens*, aflatoxins, wheat cover smut, and ricin. Field trials were conducted with *Bacillus subtilis* (a simulant for anthrax), botulinum toxin, and aflatoxin.

Biological agents were tested in various delivery systems, including rockets, aerial bombs, and spray tanks. In December 1990, the Iraqis filled 100 R400 bombs with botulinum toxin, 50 with anthrax, and 16 with aflatoxin. In addition, 13 Al Hussein (SCUD) warheads were filled with botulinum toxin, 10 with anthrax, and 2 with aflatoxin. These weapons were deployed in January 1991 to four locations. In all, Iraq produced 19,000 liters of concentrated botulinum toxin (nearly 10,000 liters filled into munitions), 8,500 liters of concentrated anthrax (6,500 liters filled into munitions) and 2,200 liters of aflatoxin (1,580 liters filled into munitions).

The threat of biological warfare has increased in the last two decades, with a number of countries working on the offensive use of these agents. The extensive program of the former Soviet Union is now primarily under the control of Russia. Former Russian president Boris Yeltsin stated that he would put an end to further offensive biological research; however, the degree to which the program was scaled back is not known. Recent revelations from a senior BW program manager who defected from Russia in 1992 outlined a remarkably robust biological warfare program, which included active research into genetic engineering, binary biologicals and chimeras, and industrial capacity to produce agents. There is also growing concern that the smallpox virus, now stored in only two laboratories at the CDC in Atlanta and the Institute for Viral Precautions in Moscow, may be in other countries around the globe.

There is intense concern in the West about the possibility of proliferation or enhancement of offensive programs in countries hostile to the western democracies, due to the potential hiring of expatriate Russian scientists. It was reported in January 1998 that Iraq had sent about a dozen scientists involved in BW research to Libya to help that country develop a biological warfare complex disguised as a medical facility in the Tripoli area. In a report issued in November 1997, Secretary of Defense William Cohen singled out Libya, Iraq, Iran, and Syria as countries "aggressively seeking" nuclear, biological, and chemical weapons.

Finally, there is an increasing amount of concern over the possibility of the terrorist use of biological agents to threaten either military or civilian populations. There have been cases of extremist groups trying to obtain microorganisms that could be used as biological weapons. The 1995 sarin nerve agent attack in the Tokyo subway system raised awareness that terrorist organizations could potentially acquire or develop WMD's for use against civilian populations. Subsequent investigations revealed the organization had attempted to release botulinum toxins and anthrax on several occasions. The Department of Defense has been leading a federal effort to train the first responders in 120 American cities to be prepared to act in case of a domestic terrorist incident involving WMD. The program will be handed over to the Department of Justice on October 1, 2000. In the past two years, first responders, public health and medical personnel, and law enforcement agencies have dealt with the exponential increase in biological weapons hoaxes around the country.

Certainly the threat of biological weapons being used against U.S. military forces and civilians is broader and more likely in various geographic scenarios than at any point in our history. Therefore, awareness of this potential threat and education of our leaders, medical care providers, public health officials, and law enforcement personnel on how to combat it are crucial.

DISTINGUISHING BETWEEN NATURAL AND INTENTIONAL DISEASE OUTBREAKS

With a covert biological agent attack, the most likely first indicator of an event would be an increased number of patients presenting with clinical features caused by the disseminated disease agent. Therefore, health care providers must use epidemiology to detect and respond rapidly to a biological agent attack.

A sound epidemiologic investigation of a disease outbreak, whether natural or human-engineered, will assist medical personnel in identifying the pathogen, as well as instituting the appropriate medical interventions. Documenting the affected population, possible routes of exposure, signs and symptoms of disease, along with rapid laboratory identification of the causative agents, will greatly increase the ability to institute an appropriate medical and public health response. Good epidemiologic information can guide the appropriate follow-up of those potentially exposed, as well as assist in risk communication and responses to the media.

Many diseases caused by weaponized biological agents present with nonspecific clinical features that could be difficult to diagnose and recognize as a biological attack. The disease pattern that develops is an important factor in differentiating between a natural and a terrorist or warfare attack. Epidemiologic clues that can potentially indicate an intentional attack are listed in Table 1. While a helpful guide, it is important to remember that naturally occurring epidemics can have one or more of these characteristics and a biological attack may have none.

Once a biological attack or any outbreak of disease is suspected, the epidemiologic investigation should begin. The conduct of the investigation will not differ significantly whether or not the outbreak is intentional. The first step is to confirm that a disease outbreak has occurred. A case definition should be constructed to determine the number of cases and the attack rate. The case definition allows investigators who are separated geographically to use the same criteria when evaluating the outbreak. The use of objective criteria in the development of a case definition is very important in determining an accurate case number, as additional cases may be found and some cases may be excluded, especially as the potential exists for hysteria to be confused with actual disease. The estimated rate of illness should be compared with rates during previous years to determine if the rate constitutes a deviation from the norm.

Once the attack rate has been determined, the outbreak can be described by time, place, and person. These data will provide crucial information in determining the potential source of the outbreak. The epidemic curve is calculated based on cases over time. In a point-source outbreak, which is most likely in a biological attack or terrorism situation, the early parts of the epidemic curve will tend to be compressed compared with propagated outbreaks. The peak may be in a matter of days or even hours. Later phases of the curve may also help determine if the disease appears to spread from person to person, which can be extremely important for determining effective disease control measures.

Well before any event, public health authorities must implement surveillance systems so they can recognize patterns of nonspecific syndromes that could indicate the early manifestations of a biological warfare attack. The system must be timely, sensitive, specific, and practical. To recognize any unusual changes in disease occurrence, surveillance of background disease activity should be ongoing, and any variation should be followed up promptly with a directed examination of the facts regarding the change.

It is important to remember that recognition of and preparation for a biological attack is similar to that for any disease outbreak, but the surveillance, response, and other demands on resources would likely be of an unparalleled intensity. A strong public health infrastructure with epidemiologic investigation capability, practical training programs, and preparedness plans are essential to prevent and control disease outbreaks, whether they are naturally occurring or otherwise.

Table 1. Epidemiologic Clues of a Biologic Warfare or Terrorist Attack
- The presence of a large epidemic with a similar disease or syndrome, especially in a discrete population
- Many cases of unexplained diseases or deaths
- More severe disease than is usually expected for a specific pathogen or failure to respond to standard therapy

- Unusual routes of exposure for a pathogen, such as the inhalational route for diseases that normally occur through other exposures
- A disease that is unusual for a given geographic area or transmission season
- Disease normally transmitted by a vector that is not present in the local area
- Multiple simultaneous or serial epidemics of different diseases in the same population
- A single case of disease by an uncommon agent (smallpox, some viral hemorrhagic fevers)
- A disease that is unusual for an age group
- Unusual strains or variants of organisms or antimicrobial resistance patterns different from those circulating
- Similar genetic type among agents isolated from distinct sources at different times or locations
- Higher attack rates in those exposed in certain areas, such as inside a building if released indoors, or lower rates in those inside a sealed building if released outside
- Disease outbreaks of the same illness occurring in noncontiguous areas
- A disease outbreak with zoonotic impact
- Intelligence of a potential attack, claims by a terrorist or aggressor of a release, and discovery of munitions or tampering

TEN STEPS IN THE MANAGEMENT OF BIOLOGICAL CASUALTIES ON THE BATTLEFIELD

Military personnel on the modern battlefield face a wide range of conventional and unconventional threats. Compared to conventional, chemical, and nuclear weapon threats, biological weapons are, perhaps, somewhat unique in their ability to cause confusion, disruption and panic. It is useful for medical care providers to understand the factors (Table 1) that account for this ability and for the difficulties they would be expected to face in dealing with biological casualties.

Potential for massive numbers of casualties
Ability to produce lengthy illnesses requiring prolonged and extensive care
Ability of certain agents to spread via contagion
Paucity of adequate detection systems
Diminished role for self-aid & buddy aid, thereby increasing sense of helplessness
Presence of an incubation period, enabling victims to disperse widely
Ability to produce non-specific symptoms, complicating diagnosis
Ability to mimic endemic infectious diseases, further complicating diagnosis

Table 1. Characteristics of Biological Weapons and Warfare

In light of these somewhat unique properties of biological weapons, medical personnel will require a firm understanding of certain key elements of biological defense in order to manage effectively the consequences of a biological attack amidst the confusion expected on the modern battlefield. Understanding the behavior, pathogenesis, modes of transmission, diagnostic modalities, and available treatment options for each of the potential agents thus becomes imperative. Acquiring such an understanding is relatively straightforward once the identity of the agent is known; many references (FM 8-9, FM 8-33, FM 8-284), including this handbook, exist to assist medical personnel in agent-based therapy. Proper and thorough evaluation and management of a potential biological attack, before a causative agent is identified, however, is likely to be complex and problematic. For this reason, we recommend a ten-step process to guide medical personnel in such evaluation and management.

I. **Maintain an index of suspicion.** The health-care provider on the modern battlefield must first possess a high index of suspicion regarding the potential employment of biological weapons. This is due to the fact that, with many of the biological warfare (BW) diseases, very early treatment is mandatory if patients are to be salvaged. Anthrax, botulism, plague, and smallpox are readily prevented if patients are provided proper antibiotics, antisera, and/or immunization promptly following exposure. Conversely, all of these diseases may prove fatal if therapy or prophylaxis is delayed until classic symptoms develop. Unfortunately, symptoms in the early, or prodromal, phase of illness are non-specific, making diagnosis difficult. Moreover, many potential BW diseases, such as Brucellosis, Q-fever, and Venezuelan Equine Encephalitis (VEE), may never present as more than non-specific febrile illnesses. Without a high index of suspicion, it is unlikely that the battlefield provider, especially at lower echelons, removed from sophisticated laboratory and preventive medicine resources, will promptly arrive at a proper diagnosis and institute appropriate therapy.

II. Protect Thyself. Before medical personnel approach a potential biological casualty, they must first take steps to protect themselves. These steps may involve a combination of physical, chemical, and immunologic forms of protection. On the battlefield, physical protection typically consists of a protective mask. Designed primarily with chemical vapor hazards in mind, the M-40 series mask certainly provides adequate protection against all inhalational BW threats. In fact, a HEPA-filter (or even a simple surgical) mask will afford adequate protection against BW (although not against chemical) threats. Chemical protection refers, in general, to the pre- and/or post-exposure administration of antibiotics; such strategies are discussed on an agent-specific basis elsewhere in this book. Immunologic protection principally involves active immunization and, in the present climate, applies mainly to protection against anthrax. Again, specific immunization strategies are discussed throughout this book.

III. Assess the Patient. This initial assessment is somewhat analogous to the primary survey of ATLS management. As such, airway adequacy should be assessed and breathing and circulation problems addressed before attention is given to specific management. The initial assessment is conducted before decontamination is accomplished and should thus be brief. Historical information of potential interest to the clinician might include information about illnesses in other unit members, the presence of unusual munitions, food and water procurement sources, vector exposure, immunization history, travel history, occupational duties, and MOPP status. Physical exam at this point should concentrate on the pulmonary and neuromuscular systems, as well as unusual dermatologic and vascular findings.

IV. Decontaminate as Appropriate. Decontamination plays a very important role in the approach to chemical casualty management. The incubation period of biological agents, however, makes it unlikely that victims of a BW attack will present for medical care until days after an attack. At this point, the need for decontamination is minimal or non-existent. In those rare cases where decontamination is warranted, simple soap and water bathing will usually suffice. Certainly, standard military decontamination solutions (such as hypochlorite), typically employed in cases of chemical agent contamination, would be effective against all biological agents. In fact, even 0.1% bleach reliably kills anthrax spores, the hardiest of biological agents. Routine use of caustic substances, especially on human skin, however, is rarely warranted following a biological attack. More information on decontamination is included elsewhere in this text.

V. Establish a Diagnosis. With decontamination (where warranted) accomplished, a more thorough attempt to establish a diagnosis can be carried out. This attempt, somewhat analogous, to the secondary survey used in the ATLS approach, should involve a combination of clinical, epidemiologic, and laboratory examinations. The amount of expertise and support available to the clinician will vary at each echelon of care. At higher echelons, a full range of laboratory capabilities should enable definitive diagnosis. At lower echelons, every attempt should be made to obtain diagnostic specimens from representative patients and forward these through laboratory channels. Nasal swabs (important for culture and PCR, even if the clinician is unsure *which* organisms to assay for), blood cultures, serum, sputum cultures, blood and urine for toxin analysis, throat swabs, and environmental samples should be considered.

Respiratory Casualties	
Rapid-Onset	**Delayed-Onset**
Nerve Agents	Inhalational Anthrax
Cyanide	Pneumonic Plague
Mustard	Pneumonic Tularemia
Lewisite	Q Fever
Phosgene	SEB Inhalation
SEB Inhalation	Ricin Inhalation
	Mustard
	Lewisite
	Phosgene
Neurological Casualties	
Rapid-Onset	**Delayed-Onset**
Nerve Agents	Botulism-peripheral symptoms
Cyanide	VEE-CNS symptoms

Table 2. Diagnostic Matrix: Chemical & Biological Casualties.

While awaiting laboratory confirmation, a diagnosis must be made on clinical grounds. Access, at higher echelons, to infectious disease, preventive medicine, and other specialists, can assist in this process. At lower echelons, the clinician should, at the very least, be familiar with the concept of syndromic diagnosis. Chemical and biological warfare diseases can be generally divided into those that present "immediately" with little or no incubation or latent period (principally the chemical agents) and those with a considerable delay in presentation (principally the biological agents). Moreover, BW diseases are likely to present as one of a limited number of clinical syndromes. Plague, Tularemia, and SEB disease all may present as pneumonia. Botulism and VEE may present with peripheral and central neuromuscular findings, respectively. This allows the construction of a simple diagnostic matrix as shown in Table 2. Even syndromic diagnosis, however, is complicated by the fact that many BW diseases (VEE, Q-Fever, Brucellosis) may present simply as undifferentiated febrile illnesses. Moreover, other diseases (Anthrax, Plague, Tularemia, Smallpox) have undifferentiated febrile prodromes.

VI. Render Prompt Treatment. Unfortunately, it is precisely in the prodromal phase of many diseases that therapy is most likely to be effective. For this reason, empiric therapy of pneumonia or undifferentiated febrile illness on the battlefield might be indicated under certain circumstances. Table 3 is constructed by eliminating from consideration those diseases for which definitive therapy is not warranted, not available, or not critical. Empiric treatment of respiratory casualties (patients with undifferentiated febrile illnesses who might have prodromal anthrax, plague, or tularemia would be managed in a similar manner) might then be entertained. Doxycycline, for example, is effective against most strains of *B. anthracis, Y. pestis,* and *F. tularensis,* as well as against *C. burnetii*, and the *Brucellae*. Other tetracyclines and fluoroquinolones might also be considered. Keep in mind that such therapy is, in no way, a substitute for a careful and thorough diagnostic evaluation, when battlefield conditions permit such an evaluation.

Respiratory Casualties	
Rapid-Onset	**Delayed-Onset**
Cyanide	Inhalational Anthrax
	Pneumonic Plague
	Pneumonic Tularemia
Neurological Casualties	
Rapid-Onset	**Delayed-Onset**
Nerve Agents	Botulism

Table 3. CW & BW Diseases Potentially Requiring Prompt Empiric Therapy.

VII. Practice Good Infection Control. Standard precautions provide adequate protection against most infectious diseases, including those potentially employed in BW. Anthrax, Tularemia, Brucellosis, Glanders, Q-Fever, VEE, and the Toxin-Mediated diseases are not generally contagious, and victims can be safely managed using standard precautions. Such precautions should be familiar to all clinicians. Under certain circumstances, however, one of three forms of transmission-based precautions would be warranted. Smallpox victims should, wherever possible, be managed using airborne precautions. Pneumonic Plague warrants the use of droplet precautions, and certain VHFs require contact precautions.

VIII. Alert the Proper Authorities. In any military context, the command should immediately be apprised of casualties suspected due to chemical or biological agents. The clinical laboratory should also be notified. This will enable laboratory personnel to take proper precautions when handling specimens and will also permit the optimal use of various diagnostic modalities. Chemical Corps and Preventive Medicine personnel should be contacted to assist in the delineation of contaminated areas and the search for further victims.

IX. Assist in the Epidemiologic Investigation. All health care providers require a basic understanding of epidemiologic principles. Even under austere conditions, a rudimentary epidemiologic investigation may assist in diagnosis and in the discovery of additional BW victims. Clinicians should, at the very least, query patients about potential exposures, ill unit members, food/water sources, unusual munitions or spray devices, vector exposures, and develop a line listing of potential cases. Such early discovery might, in turn, permit post-exposure prophylaxis, thereby avoiding excess morbidity and mortality. Preventive medicine officers, field sanitation personnel, epidemiology technicians, environmental science officers, and veterinary officers are all available to assist the clinician in conducting an epidemiologic investigation.

X. Maintain Proficiency and Spread the Gospel. Fortunately, the threat of BW has remained a theoretical one for most medical personnel. Inability to practice casualty management, however, can lead to a rapid loss of skills and knowledge. It is imperative that the medic maintains proficiency in dealing with this low probability, but high consequence problem. This can be done, in part, by availing oneself of several resources.

22

The OTSG (www.nbc-med.org) and USAMRIID (www.usamriid.army.mil) Web Sites provide a wealth of information, including the text of this handbook. Annual satellite television broadcasts, sponsored by USAMRIID, provide in-depth discussion and training in medical biodefense as well. A CD-ROM training aid has been developed, and a new field manual (Army FM 8-284) summarizes BW disease management recommendations. Finally, medical personnel, once aware of the threat and trained to deal with it, must ensure that other personnel in their units receive training as well. It is only through ongoing training that you will be ready to deal with the threat posed by biological weapons. By familiarizing yourself with the contents of this handbook, you have taken a large step towards such readiness.

BACTERIAL AGENTS

Bacteria are unicellular organisms. They vary in shape and size from spherical cells - cocci - with a diameter of 0.5-1.0 µm (micrometer), to long rod-shaped organisms - bacilli - which may be from 1-5 µm in size. Chains of bacilli may exceed 50 µm in length. The shape of the bacterial cell is determined by the rigid cell wall. The interior of the cell contains the nuclear material (DNA), cytoplasm, and cell membrane, that are necessary for the life of the bacterium. Many bacteria also have glycoproteins on their outer surfaces which aid in bacterial attachment to cell surface receptors. Under special circumstances some types of bacteria can transform into spores. The spore of the bacterial cell is more resistant to cold, heat, drying, chemicals and radiation than the vegetative bacterium itself. Spores are a dormant form of the bacterium and, like the seeds of plants, they can germinate when conditions are favorable.

The term rickettsia generally applies to very small, gram-negative coccobacillary organisms of the genera *Rickettsia* and *Coxiella*. Rickettsiae are unique from classical bacteria in their inability to grow (with rare exceptions) in the absence of a living host cell, but many are susceptible to treatment with antibiotics.

Bacteria generally cause disease in human beings and animals by one of two mechanisms: by invading host tissues, and by producing poisons (toxins). Many pathogenic bacteria utilize both mechanisms. The diseases they produce often respond to specific therapy with antibiotics. It is important to distinguish between the disease-causing organism and the name of the disease it causes (in parentheses below). This manual covers several of the bacteria or rickettsiae considered to be potential BW threat agents: *Bacillus anthracis* (Anthrax), *Brucella* spp. (Brucellosis), *Burkholderia mallei* (Glanders), *Burholderia pseudomallei* (melioidosis), *Yersinia pestis* (Plague), *Francisella tularensis* (Tularemia), and *Coxiella burnetii* (Q Fever).

ANTHRAX

SUMMARY

Signs and Symptoms: Incubation period is generally 1-6 days, although longer periods have been noted. Fever, malaise, fatigue, cough and mild chest discomfort progresses to severe respiratory distress with dyspnea, diaphoresis, stridor, cyanosis, and shock. Death typically occurs within 24-36 hours after onset of severe symptoms.

Diagnosis: Physical findings are non-specific. A widened mediastinum may be seen on CXR in later stages of illness. The organism is detectable by Gram stain of the blood and by blood culture late in the course of illness.

Treatment: Although effectiveness may be limited after symptoms are present, high dose antibiotic treatment with penicillin, ciprofloxacin, or doxycycline should be undertaken. Supportive therapy may be necessary.

Prophylaxis: Oral ciprofloxacin or doxycycline for known or imminent exposure. An FDA-licensed vaccine is available. Vaccine schedule is 0.5 ml SC at 0, 2, 4 weeks, then 6, 12, and 18 months (primary series), followed by annual boosters.

Isolation and Decontamination: Standard precautions for healthcare workers. After an invasive procedure or autopsy is performed, the instruments and area used should be thoroughly disinfected with a sporicidal agent (hypochlorite).

OVERVIEW

Bacillus anthracis, the causative agent of Anthrax, is a gram-positive, sporulating rod. The spores are the usual infective form. Anthrax is primarily a zoonotic disease of herbivores, with cattle, sheep, goats, and horses being the usual domesticated animal hosts, but other animals may be infected. Humans generally contract the disease when handling contaminated hair, wool, hides, flesh, blood and excreta of infected animals and from manufactured products such as bone meal. Infection is introduced through scratches or abrasions of the skin, wounds, inhalation of spores, eating insufficiently cooked infected meat, or by biting flies. The primary concern for intentional infection by this organism is through inhalation after aerosol dissemination of spores. All human populations are susceptible. The spores are very stable and may remain viable for many years in soil and water. They resist sunlight for varying periods.

HISTORY AND SIGNIFICANCE

Anthrax spores were weaponized by the United States in the 1950's and 1960's before the old U.S. offensive program was terminated. Other countries have weaponized this agent or are suspected of doing so. Anthrax bacteria are easy to cultivate and spore production is readily induced. Moreover, the spores are highly resistant to sunlight, heat and disinfectants - properties which could be advantageous when choosing a bacterial weapon. Iraq admitted to a United Nations inspection team in August of 1991 that it had performed research on the offensive use of *B. anthracis* prior to the Persian Gulf War, and in 1995 Iraq admitted to weaponizing anthrax. A recent defector from the former Soviet Union's biological weapons program revealed that the Soviets had produced anthrax in ton quantities for use as a weapon. This agent could be produced in either a wet or dried form, stabilized for weaponization by an adversary and delivered as an aerosol cloud either from a line source such as an aircraft flying upwind of friendly positions, or as a point source from a spray device. Coverage of a large ground area could also be theoretically facilitated by multiple spray bomblets disseminated from a missile warhead at a predetermined height above the ground.

CLINICAL FEATURES

Anthrax presents as three somewhat distinct clinical syndromes in humans: cutaneous, inhalational, and gastrointestinal disease. The cutaneous form (also referred to as a malignant pustule) occurs most frequently on the hands and forearms of persons working with infected livestock. It begins as a papule followed by formation of a fluid-filled vesicle. The vesicle typically dries and forms a coal-black scab (eschar), hence the term anthrax (from the Greek for coal). This local infection can occasionally disseminate into a fatal systemic infection. Gastrointestinal anthrax is rare in humans, and is contracted by the ingestion of insufficiently cooked meat from infected animals. Endemic inhalational anthrax, known as Woolsorters' disease, is also a rare infection contracted by inhalation of the spores. It occurs mainly among workers in an industrial setting handling infected hides, wool, and furs. In man, the mortality of untreated cutaneous anthrax ranges up to 25 per cent; in inhalational and intestinal cases, the case fatality rate is almost 100 percent.

DIAGNOSIS

After an incubation period of 1-6 days,* presumably dependent upon the dose and strain of inhaled organisms, the onset of inhalation anthrax is gradual and nonspecific. Fever, malaise, and fatigue may be present, sometimes in association with a nonproductive cough and mild chest discomfort. These initial symptoms are often followed by a short period of improvement (hours to 2-3 days), followed by the abrupt development of severe respiratory distress with dyspnea, diaphoresis, stridor, and cyanosis. Septicemia, shock and death usually follow within 24-36 hours after the onset of respiratory distress. Physical findings are typically non-specific, especially in the early phase of the disease. The chest X-ray may reveal a widened mediastinum ± pleural effusions late in the disease in about 55% of the cases, but typically is without infiltrates. Pneumonia generally does not occur; therefore, organisms are not typically seen in the sputum. *Bacillus anthracis* will be detectable by Gram stain of the blood and by blood culture with routine media, but often not until late in the course of the illness. Approximately 50% of cases are accompanied by hemorrhagic meningitis, and therefore organisms may also be identified in cerebrospinal fluid. Only vegetative encapsulated bacilli are present during infection. Spores are not found within the body unless it is open to ambient air. Studies of inhalation anthrax in non-human primates (rhesus monkey) showed that bacilli and toxin appear in the blood late on day 2 or early on day 3 post-exposure. Toxin production parallels the appearance of bacilli in the blood and tests are available to rapidly detect the toxin. Concurrently with the appearance of anthrax, the WBC count becomes elevated and remains so until death.

*During an outbreak of inhalational anthrax in the Soviet Union in 1979, persons are reported to have become ill up to 6 weeks after an aerosol release occurred.

MEDICAL MANAGEMENT

Almost all inhalational anthrax cases in which treatment was begun after patients were significantly symptomatic have been fatal, regardless of treatment. Penicillin has been regarded as the treatment of choice, with 2 million units given intravenously every 2 hours. Tetracyclines and erythromycin have been recommended in penicillin allergic patients. The vast majority of naturally-occurring anthrax strains are sensitive *in vitro* to penicillin. However, penicillin-resistant strains exist naturally, and one has been recovered from a fatal human case. Moreover, it might not be difficult for an adversary to induce resistance to penicillin, tetracyclines, erythromycin, and many other antibiotics through laboratory manipulation of organisms. All naturally occurring strains tested to date have been sensitive to erythromycin, chloramphenicol, gentamicin, and ciprofloxacin. In the absence of antibiotic sensitivity data, empiric intravenous antibiotic treatment should be instituted at the earliest signs of disease. Military policy (FM 8-284) currently recommends ciprofloxacin (400 mg IV q 12 hrs) or doxycycline (200 mg IV load, followed by 100 mg IV q 12 hrs) as initial therapy, with penicillin (4 million U IV q 4 hours) as an alternative once sensitivity data is available. Published recommendations from a public health consensus panel recommends ciprofloxacin as initial therapy. Therapy may then be tailored once antibiotic sensitivity is available to penicillin G or doxycycline. Recommended treatment duration is 60 days, and should be changed to oral therapy as clinical condition improves. Supportive therapy for shock, fluid volume deficit, and adequacy of airway may all be needed.

Standard Precautions are recommended for patient care. There is no evidence of direct person-to-person spread of disease from inhalational anthrax. After an invasive procedure or autopsy, the instruments and area used should be thoroughly disinfected with a sporicidal agent. Iodine can be used, but must be used at disinfectant strengths, as antiseptic-strength iodophors are not usually sporicidal. Chlorine, in the form of sodium or calcium hypochlorite, can also be used, but with the caution that the activity of hypochlorites is greatly reduced in the presence of organic material.

PROPHYLAXIS

Vaccine: A licensed vaccine (Anthrax Vaccine Adsorbed) is derived from sterile culture fluid supernatant taken from an attenuated strain. Therefore, the vaccine does not contain live or dead organisms. The vaccination series consists of six 0.5 ml doses SC at 0, 2, and 4 weeks, then 6, 12 and 18 months, followed by yearly boosters. A human efficacy trial in mill workers demonstrated protection against cutaneous anthrax. There is insufficient data to know its efficacy against inhalational anthrax in humans, although studies in rhesus monkeys indicate that good protection can be afforded after only two doses (15 days apart) for up to 2 years. However, it should be emphasized that the vaccine series should be completed according to the licensed 6 dose primary series. As with all vaccines, the degree of protection depends upon the magnitude of the challenge dose; vaccine-induced protection could presumably be overwhelmed by extremely high spore challenge. Current military policy is to restart the primary vaccine series only if greater than two years elapses between the first and second doses. For all other missed doses, administer the missed dose ASAP and reset the timeline for the series based on the most recent dose.

Contraindications for use of this vaccine include hypersensitivity reaction to a previous dose of vaccine and age < 18 or > 65. Reasons for temporary deferment of the vaccine include pregnancy, active infection with fever, or a course of immune suppressing drugs such as steroids. Reactogenicity is mild to moderate. Up to 30 percent of recipients may experience mild discomfort at the inoculation site for up to 72 hours (e.g., tenderness, erythema, edema, pruritus), fewer experience moderate reactions, while less than 1 percent may experience more severe local reactions, potentially limiting use of the arm for 1-2 days. Modest systemic reactions (e.g., myalgia, malaise, low-grade fever) are uncommon, and severe systemic reactions such as anaphylaxis, which precludes additional vaccination, are rare. The vaccine should be stored between 2-6° C (refrigerator temperature, not frozen).

Antibiotics: Both Military doctrine and a public health consensus panel recommend prophylaxis with ciprofloxacin (500 mg po bid) as the first-line medication in a situation with anthrax as the presumptive agent. Ciprofloxacin recently became the first medication approved by the FDA for prophylaxis after exposure to a biological weapon (anthrax). Alternatives are doxycycline (100 mg po bid) or amoxicillin (500mg po q 8 hours), if the strain is susceptible. Should an attack be confirmed as anthrax, antibiotics should be continued for at least 4 weeks in all those exposed, and until all those exposed have received three doses of the vaccine. Those who have already received three doses within 6 months of exposure should continue with their routine vaccine schedule. In the absence of vaccine, chemoprophylaxis should continue for at least 60 days. Upon discontinuation of antibiotics, patients should be closely observed. If clinical signs of anthrax occur, empiric therapy for anthrax is indicated, pending etiologic diagnosis. Optimally, patients should have medical care available upon discontinuation of antibiotics, from a fixed medical care facility with intensive care capabilities and infectious disease consultants.

BRUCELLOSIS

SUMMARY

Signs and Symptoms: Illness, when manifest, typically presents with fever, headache, myalgias, arthralgias, back pain, sweats, chills, and generalized malaise. Other manifestations include depression, mental status changes, and osteoarticular findings (ie. Sacroiliitis, vertebral osteomyelitis). Fatalities are uncommon.

Diagnosis: Diagnosis requires a high index of suspicion, since many infections present as non-specific febrile illnesses or are asymptomatic. Laboratory diagnosis can be made by blood culture with prolonged incubation. Bone marrow cultures produce a higher yield. Confirmation requires phage-typing, oxidative metabolism, or genotyping procedures. ELISA, followed by Western blot are available.

Treatment: Antibiotic therapy with doxycycline + rifampin or doxycycline in combination with other medications for six weeks is usually sufficient in most cases. More prolonged regimens may be required for patients with complications of meningoencephalitis, endocarditis, or osteomyelitis.

Prophylaxis: There is no human vaccine available against brucellosis, although animal vaccines exist. Chemoprophylaxis is not recommended after possible exposure to endemic disease. Treatment should be considered for high-risk exposure to the veterinary vaccine, inadvertent laboratory exposure, or confirmed biological warfare exposure.

Isolation and Decontamination: Standard precautions are appropriate for healthcare workers. Person-to-person transmission has been reported via tissue transplantation and sexual contact. Environmental decontamination can be accomplished with a 0.5% hypochlorite solution.

OVERVIEW

Brucellosis is one of the world's most important veterinary diseases, and is caused by infection with one of six species of *Brucellae,* a group of gram-negative cocco-baccillary facultative intracellular pathogens. In animals, brucellosis primarily involves the reproductive tract, causing septic abortion and orchitis, which, in turn, can result in sterility. Consequently, brucellosis is a disease of great potential economic impact in the animal husbandry industry. Four species (*B. abortus, B. melitensis, B. suis*, and, rarely, *B. canis*) are pathogenic in humans. Infections in abattoir and laboratory workers suggest that the *Brucellae* are highly infectious via the aerosol route. It is estimated that inhalation of only 10 to 100 bacteria is sufficient to cause disease in man. Brucellosis has a low mortality rate (5% of untreated cases), with rare deaths caused by endocarditis or meningitis. Also, given that the disease has a relatively long and variable incubation period (5-60 days), and that many naturally occurring infections are asymptomatic, its usefulness as a weapon may be diminished. Large aerosol doses, however, may shorten the incubation period and increase the clinical attack rate, and the disease is relatively prolonged, incapacitating, and disabling in its natural form.

HISTORY AND SIGNIFICANCE

Marston described the manifestations of disease caused by *B. melitensis* ("Mediterranean gastric remittent fever") among British soldiers on Malta during the Crimean War. Work by the Mediterranean Fever

Commission identified goats as the source, and restrictions on the ingestion of unpasteurized goat milk products soon decreased the number of brucellosis cases among military personnel.

In 1954, *Brucella suis* became the first agent weaponized by the United States at Pine Bluff Arsenal when its offensive BW program was active. Brucella weapons, along with the remainder of the U.S. biological arsenal, were destroyed in 1969, when the offensive program was disbanded.

Human brucellosis is now an uncommon disease in the United States, with an annual incidence of 0.5 cases per 100,000 population. Most cases are associated with the ingestion of unpasteurized dairy products, or with abattoir and veterinary work. The disease is, however, highly endemic in southwest Asia (annual incidence as high as 128 cases per 100,000 in some areas of Kuwait), thus representing a hazard to military personnel stationed in that theater.

CLINICAL FEATURES

Brucellosis, also known as "undulant fever", typically presents as a nonspecific febrile illness resembling influenza. Fever, headache, myalgias, arthralgias, back pain, sweats, chills, generalized weakness, and malaise are common complaints. Cough and pleuritic chest pain occurs In up to twenty percent of cases, but acute pneumonitis is unusual, and pulmonary symptoms may not correlate with radiographic findings. The chest x-ray is often normal, but may show lung abscesses, single or miliary nodules, bronchopneumonia, enlarged hilar lymph nodes, and pleural effusions. Gastrointestinal symptoms (anorexia, nausea, vomiting, diarrhea and constipation) occur in up to 70 percent of adult cases, but less frequently in children. Ileitis, colitis, and granulomatous or mononuclear infiltrative hepatitis may occur, with hepato- and spleno-megaly present in 45-63 percent of cases.

Lumbar pain and tenderness can occur in up to 60% of brucellosis cases and are sometimes due to various osteoarticular infections of the axial skeleton. Vertebral osteomyelitis, intervertebral disc space infection, paravertebral abscess, and sacroiliac infection occur in a minority of cases, but may be a cause of chronic symptoms. Consequently, persistent fever following therapy or the prolonged presence of significant musculoskeletal complaints should prompt CT or MR imaging. [99m]Technetium and [67]Gallium scans are also reasonably sensitive means for detecting sacroiliitis and other axial skeletal infections. Joint involvement in brucellosis may vary from pain to joint immobility and effusion. While the sacroiliac joints are most commonly involved, peripheral joints (notably, hips, knees, and ankles) may also be affected. Meningitis complicates a small minority of brucellosis cases, and encephalitis, peripheral neuropathy, radiculoneuropathy and meningovascular syndromes have also been observed in rare instances. Behavioral disturbances and psychoses appear to occur out of proportion to the height of fever, or to the amount of overt CNS disease. This raises questions about an ill-defined neurotoxic component of brucellosis.

DIAGNOSIS

Because most cases of brucellosis present as non-specific febrile illnesses, diagnostic hallmarks are lacking and the disease is often unsuspected. Maintenance of a high index of suspicion is thus critical if one is to firmly establish a diagnosis of brucellosis. A history of animal contact, consumption of unpasteurized dairy and goat-milk products, or travel to areas where such consumption is common, should prompt consideration of endemic brucellosis as a diagnosis. The leukocyte count in brucellosis patients is usually normal but may be low; anemia and thrombocytopenia may also occur. Blood and bone marrow cultures during the acute febrile phase of illness yield the organism in 15-70% and 92% of cases, respectively. A biphasic culture method for blood (Castaneda bottle) may improve the chances of isolation. Clinical laboratories should always be alerted if a diagnosis of brucellosis is suspected. This permits the use of selective isolation media and the implementation of Biosafety Level-3 (BSL-3) safety precautions. A serum agglutination test (SAT) is available to detect both IgM and IgG antibodies; a titer of 1:160 or greater is indicative of active disease. ELISA and PCR methods are becoming more widely utilized.

MEDICAL MANAGEMENT

Standard precautions are adequate in managing brucellosis patients, as the disease is not generally transmissible from person-to-person. As noted previously, BSL-3 practices should be used when handling suspected brucella cultures in the laboratory because of the danger of inhalation in this setting.

Oral antibiotic therapy alone is sufficient in most cases of brucellosis. Exceptions involve uncommon cases of localized disease, where surgical intervention may be required (e.g., valve replacement for endocarditis). A combination of Doxycycline 200 mg/d PO + Rifampin 600 mg/d PO is generally recommended. Both drugs should be administered for six weeks. Doxycycline 200 mg/d PO for six weeks in combination with two weeks of Streptomycin (1 g/d IM) is an acceptable alternative. Regimens involving Doxycycline + Gentamicin, TMP/SMX + Gentamicin, and Ofloxacin + Rifampin have also been studied and shown effective. Long-term triple-drug therapy with rifampin, a tetracycline, and an aminoglycoside is recommended by some experts for patients with meningoencephalitis or endocarditis.

PROPHYLAXIS

The risk of endemic brucellosis can be diminished by the avoidance of unpasteurized goat-milk and dairy products, especially while travelling in areas where veterinary brucellosis remains common. Live animal vaccines are used widely, and have eliminated brucellosis from most domestic animal herds in the United States, although no licensed human brucellosis vaccine is available.

Chemoprophylaxis is not generally recommended following possible exposure to endemic disease. A 3-6 week course of therapy (with one of the regimens discussed above) should be considered following a high-risk exposure to veterinary vaccine (such as a needle-stick injury), inadvertent exposure in a laboratory, or exposure in a biological warfare context.

GLANDERS AND MELIOIDOSIS

SUMMARY

Signs and Symptoms: Incubation period ranges from 10-14 days after inhalation. Onset of symptoms may be abrupt or gradual. Inhalational exposure produces fever (common in excess of 102 F.), rigors, sweats, myalgias, headache, pleuritic chest pain, cervical adenopathy, hepatosplenomegaly, and generalized papular / pustular eruptions. Acute pulmonary disease can progress and result in bacteremia and acute septicemic disease. Both diseases are almost always fatal without treatment.

Diagnosis: Methylene blue or Wright stain of exudates may reveal scant small bacilli with a safety-pin bipolar appearance. Standard cultures can be used to identify both *B. mallei* and *B. pseudomallei*. CXR may show miliary lesions, small multiple lung abscesses, or infiltrates involving upper lungs, with consolidation and cavitation. Leukocyte counts may be normal or elevated. Serologic tests can help confirm diagnosis, but low titers or negative serology does not exclude the diagnosis.

Treatment: Therapy will vary with the type and severity of the clinical presentation. Patients with localized disease, may be managed with oral antibiotics for a duration of 60-150 days. More severe illness may require parenteral therapy and more prolonged treatment.

Prophylaxis: Currently, no pre-exposure or post-exposure prophylaxis is available.

Isolation and Decontamination: Standard Precautions for healthcare workers. Person-to-person airborne transmission is unlikely, although secondary cases may occur through improper handling of infected secretions. Contact precautions are indicated while caring for patients with skin involvement. Environmental decontamination using a 0.5% hypochlorite solution is effective.

OVERVIEW

The causative agents of Glanders and Melioidosis are *Burkholderia mallei* and *Burkholderia pseudomallei,* respectively. Both are gram-negative bacilli with a "safety-pin" appearance on microscopic examination. Both pathogens affect domestic and wild animals, which, like humans, acquire the diseases from inhalation or contaminated injuries.

B. mallei is primarily noted for producing disease in horses, mules, and donkeys. In the past man has seldom been infected, despite frequent and often close contact with infected animals. This may be the result of exposure to low concentrations of organisms from infected sites in ill animals and because strains virulent for equids are often less virulent for man. There are four basic forms of disease in horses and man. The acute forms are more common in mules and donkeys, with death typically occurring 3 to 4 weeks after illness onset. The chronic form of the disease is more common in horses and causes generalized lymphadenopathy, multiple skin nodules that ulcerate and drain, and induration, enlargement, and nodularity of regional lymphatics on the extremities and in other areas. The lymphatic thickening and induration has been called farcy. Human cases have occurred primarily in veterinarians, horse and donkey caretakers, and abattoir workers.

B. pseudomallei is widely distributed in many tropical and subtropical regions. The disease is endemic in Southeast Asia and northern Australia. In northeastern

Thailand, *B. pseudomallei*, is one of the most common causative agents of community-acquired septicemia. Melioidosis presents in humans in several distinct forms, ranging from a subclinical illness to an overwhelming septicemia, with a 90% mortality rate and death within 24-48 hours after onset. Also, melioidosis can reactivate years after primary infection and result in chronic and life-threatening disease.

These organisms spread to man by invading the nasal, oral, and conjunctival mucous membranes, by inhalation into the lungs, and by invading abraded or lacerated skin. Aerosols from cultures have been observed to be highly infectious to laboratory workers. Biosafety level 3 containment practices are required when working with these organisms in the laboratory. Since aerosol spread is efficient, and there is no available vaccine or reliable therapy, *B. mallei* and *B. pseudomallei* have both been viewed as potential BW agents.

HISTORY AND SIGNIFICANCE

Despite the efficiency of spread in a laboratory setting, glanders has only been a sporadic disease in man, and no epidemics of human disease have been reported. There have been no naturally acquired cases of human glanders in the United States in over 61 years. Sporadic cases continue to occur in Asia, Africa, the Middle East and South America. During World War I, glanders was believed to have been spread deliberately by agents of the Central Powers to infect large numbers of Russian horses and mules on the Eastern Front. This had an effect on troop and supply convoys as well as on artillery movement, which were dependent on horses and mules. Human cases in Russia increased with the infections during and after WWI. The Japanese deliberately infected horses, civilians, and prisoners of war with *B. mallei* at the Pinfang (China) Institute during World War II. The United States studied this agent as a possible BW weapon in 1943-44 but did not weaponize it. The former Soviet Union is believed to have been interested in *B. mallei* as a potential BW agent after World War II. The low transmission rates of *B. mallei* to man from infected horses is exemplified by the fact that in China, during World War II, thirty percent of tested horses were positive for glanders, but human cases were rare. In Mongolia, 5-25% of tested animals were reactive to *B. mallei*, but no human cases were seen. *B. mallei* exists in nature only in infected susceptible hosts and is not found in water, soil, or plants.

In contrast, melioidosis is widely distributed in the soil and water in the tropics, and remains endemic in certain parts of the world, even to this day. It is one of the few genuinely tropical diseases that are well established in Southeast Asia and northern Australia. As a result of its long incubation period, it could be unknowingly imported.

B. pseudomallei was also studied by the United States as a potential BW agent, but was never weaponized. It has been reported that the former Soviet Union was experimenting with B. pseudomallei as a BW agent.

CLINICAL FEATURES

Both glanders and melioidosis may occur in an acute localized form, as an acute pulmonary infection, or as an acute fulminant, rapidly fatal, sepsis. Combinations of these syndromes may occur in human cases. Also, melioidosis may remain asymptomatic after initial acquisition, and remain quiescent for decades. However, these patients may present with active melioidosis years later, often associated with an immune-compromising state.

Aerosol infection produced by a BW weapon containing either *B. mallei* or *B. pseudomallei* could produce any of these syndromes. The incubation period ranges from 10- 14 days, depending on the inhaled dose and agent virulence. The septicemic form begins suddenly with fever, rigors, sweats, myalgias, pleuritic chest pain, granulomatous or necrotizing lesions, generalized erythroderma, jaundice, photophobia, lacrimation, and diarrhea. Physical examination may reveal fever, tachycardia, cervical adenopathy and mild hepatomegaly or splenomegaly. Blood cultures are usually negative until the patient is moribund. Mild leukocytosis with a shift to the left or leukopenia may occur.

The pulmonary form may follow inhalation or arise by hematogenous spread. Systemic symptoms as described for the septicemic form occur. Chest radiographs may show miliary nodules (0.5-1.0 cm) and/or a bilateral bronchopneumonia, segmental, or lobar pneumonia, consolidation, and cavitating lung lesions

Acute infection of the oral, nasal and/ or conjunctival mucosa can cause mucopurulent, blood streaked discharge from the nose, associated with septal and turbinate nodules and ulcerations. If systemic invasion occurs from mucosal or cutaneous lesions then a papular and / or pustular rash may occur that can be mistaken for smallpox (another possible BW agent). Evidence of dissemination of these infections includes the presence of skin pustules, abscesses of internal organs, such as liver and spleen, and multiple pulmonary lesions. This form carries a high mortality, and most patients develop rapidly progressive septic shock.

The chronic form is unlikely to be present within 14 days after a BW aerosol attack. It is characterized by cutaneous and intramuscular abscesses on the legs and arms. These lesions are associated with enlargement and induration of the regional lymph channels and nodes. The chronic form may be asymptomatic, especially with melioidosis. There have been cases associated with the development of osteomyelitis, brain abscess, and meningitis.

DIAGNOSIS

Gram stain of lesion exudates reveals small gram negative, bipolar bacteria. These stain irregularly with methylene blue or Wright's Stain. The organisms can be cultured and identified with standard bacteriological media. The addition of 1-5% glucose, 5 % glycerol, or meat infusion nutrient agar may accelerate growth. Primary isolation requires 48 hours at 37.5° C. For *B. mallei,* agglutination tests are not positive for 7-10 days, and a high background titer in normal sera (1:320 to 1:640) makes interpretation difficult. Complement fixation tests are more specific and are considered positive if the titer is equal to, or exceeds 1:20. For *B. pseudomallei,* a four fold increase in titer supports the diagnosis of melioidosis. A single titer above 1:160 with a compatible clinical picture suggests active infection. Occurrence in the absence of animal contact and / or in an epidemic, is presumptive evidence of a BW attack. Mortality will be high despite antibiotic use. In the hamster 1 to 10 organisms administered by aerosol is lethal.

MEDICAL MANAGEMENT

Standard Precautions should be used to prevent person-to-person transmission in proven or suspected cases. The recommended therapy will vary with the type and severity of the clinical presentation. The following oral regimens have been suggested for localized disease: Amoxicillin / clavulanate 60 mg/kg/day in three divided doses; Tetracycline 40 mg/kg/day in three divided doses; or Trimethoprim / sulfa (TMP 4 mg/kg/day-sulfa 20 mg/kg/day) in two divided doses. The duration of treatment should be for 60 - 150 days.

If the patient has localized disease with signs of mild toxicity, then a combination of two of the oral regimens is recommended for a duration of 30 days, followed by monotherapy with either amoxicillin / clavulanate or TMP / sulfa for 60 - 150 days. If extrapulmonary suppurative disease is present, then therapy should continue for 6-12 months. Surgical drainage of abscesses may be required.

For severe disease, parental therapy with Ceftazidime 120 mg/kg/day in three divided doses combined with TMP/sulfa (TMP 8 mg/kg/day – sulfa 40 mg/kg/day) in four divided doses for 2 weeks, followed by oral therapy for 6 months.

Other antibiotics that have been effective in experimental infection in hamsters include doxycycline, rifampin, and ciprofloxacin. The limited number of infections in humans has precluded therapeutic evaluation of most of the antibiotic agents; therefore, most antibiotic sensitivities are based on animal and *in vitro* studies. Various isolates have markedly different antibiotic sensitivities; therefore, each isolate should be tested for its own resistance pattern.

PROPHYLAXIS

Vaccine: There is no vaccine available for human use.

Antibiotics: Post-exposure chemoprophylaxis may be tried with TMP-SMX.

PLAGUE

SUMMARY

Signs and Symptoms: Pneumonic plague begins after an incubation period of 1-6 days, with high fever, chills, headache, malaise, followed by cough (often with hemoptysis), progressing rapidly to dyspnea, stridor, cyanosis, and death. Gastrointestinal symptoms are often present. Death results from respiratory failure, circulatory collapse, and a bleeding diathesis. Bubonic plague, featuring high fever, malaise, and painful lymph nodes (buboes) may progress spontaneously to the septicemic form (septic shock, thrombosis, DIC) or to the pneumonic form.

Diagnosis: Suspect plague if large numbers of previously healthy individuals develop fulminant Gram negative pneumonia, especially if hemoptysis is present. Presumptive diagnosis can be made by Gram, Wright, Giemsa or Wayson stain of blood, sputum, CSF, or lymph node aspirates. Definitive diagnosis requires culture of the organism from those sites. Immunodiagnosis is also helpful.

Treatment: Early administration of antibiotics is critical, as pneumonic plague is invariably fatal if antibiotic therapy is delayed more than 1 day after the onset of symptoms. Choose one of the following: streptomycin, gentamicin, ciprofloxacin, or doxycyclinefor 10-14 days. Chloramphenicol is the drug of choice for plague meningitis.

Prophylaxis: For asymptomatic persons exposed to a plague aerosol or to a patient with suspected pneumonic plague, give doxycycline 100 mg orally twice daily for seven days or the duration of risk of exposure plus one week. Alternative antibiotics include ciprofloxacin, tetracycline, or chloramphenicol. No vaccine is currently available for plague prophylaxis. The previously available licensed, killed vaccine was effective against bubonic plague, but not against aerosol exposure.

Isolation and Decontamination: Use Standard Precautions for bubonic plague, and Respiratory Droplet Precautions for suspected pneumonic plague. *Y. pestis* can survive in the environment for varying periods, but is susceptible to heat, disinfectants, and exposure to sunlight. Soap and water is effective if decon is needed. Take measures to prevent local disease cycles if vectors (fleas) and reservoirs (rodents) are present.

OVERVIEW

Yersinia pestis is a rod-shaped, non-motile, non-sporulating, gram-negative bacterium of the family *Enterobacteraceae.* It causes plague, a zoonotic disease of rodents (e.g., rats, mice, ground squirrels). Fleas that live on the rodents can transmit the bacteria to humans, who then suffer from the bubonic form of plague. The bubonic form may progress to the septicemic and/or pneumonic forms. Pneumonic plague would be the predominant form after a purposeful aerosol dissemination. All human populations are susceptible. Recovery from the disease is followed by temporary immunity. The organism remains viable in water, moist soil, and grains for several weeks. At near freezing temperatures, it will remain alive from months to years but is killed by 15 minutes of exposure to 55°C. It also remains viable for some time in dry sputum, flea feces, and buried bodies but is killed within several hours of exposure to sunlight.

HISTORY AND SIGNIFICANCE

The United States worked with *Y. pestis* as a potential biowarfare agent in the 1950's and 1960's before the old offensive biowarfare program was terminated, and other countries are suspected of weaponizing this organism. The former Soviet Union had more than 10 institutes and thousands of scientists who worked with plague. During World War II, Unit 731, of the Japanese Army, reportedly released plague-infected fleas from aircraft over Chinese cities. This method was cumbersome and unpredictable. The U.S.

and Soviet Union developed the more reliable and effective method of aerosolizing the organism. The interest in the terrorist potential of plague was brought to light in 1995 when Larry Wayne Harris was arrested in Ohio for the illicit procurement of a *Y. pestis* culture through the mail. The contagious nature of pneumonic plague makes it particularly dangerous as a biological weapon.

CLINICAL FEATURES

Plague normally appears in three forms in man: bubonic, septicemic, and pneumonic. The bubonic form begins after an incubation period of 2-10 days, with acute and fulminant onset of nonspecific symptoms, including high fever, malaise, headache, myalgias, and sometimes nausea and vomiting. Up to half of patients will have abdominal pain. Simultaneous with or shortly after the onset of these nonspecific symptoms, the bubo develops – a swollen, very painful, infected lymph node. Buboes are normally seen in the femoral or inguinal lymph nodes as the legs are the most commonly flea-bitten part of the adult human body. The liver and spleen are often tender and palpable. One quarter of patients will have various types of skin lesions: a pustule, vesicle, eschar or papule (containing leukocytes and bacteria) in the lymphatic drainage of the bubo, and presumably representing the site of the inoculating flea bite. Secondary septicemia is common, as greater than 80 percent of blood cultures are positive for the organism in patients with bubonic plague. However, only about a quarter of bubonic plague patients progress to clinical septicemia.

In those that do progress to secondary septicemia, as well as those presenting septicemic but without lymphadenopathy (primary septicemia), the symptoms are similar to other Gram-negative septicemias: high fever, chills, malaise, hypotension, nausea, vomiting, and diarrhea. However, plague septicemia can also produce thromboses in the acral vessels, with necrosis and gangrene, and DIC. Black necrotic appendages and more proximal purpuric lesions caused by endotoxemia are often present. Organisms can spread to the central nervous system, lungs, and elsewhere. Plague meningitis occurs in about 6% of septicemic and pneumonic cases.

Pneumonic plague is an infection of the lungs due to either inhalation of the organisms (primary pneumonic plague), or spread to the lungs from septicemia (secondary pneumonic plague). After an incubation period varying from 1 to 6 days for primary pneumonic plague (usually 2-4 days, and presumably dose-dependent), onset is acute and often fulminant. The first signs of illness include high fever, chills, headache, malaise, and myalgias, followed within 24 hours by a cough with bloody sputum. Although bloody sputum is characteristic, it can sometimes be watery or, less commonly, purulent. Gastrointestinal symptoms, including nausea, vomiting, diarrhea, and abdominal pain, may be present. Rarely, a cervical bubo might result from an inhalational exposure. The chest X-ray findings are variable, but most commonly reveal bilateral infiltrates, which may be patchy or consolidated. The pneumonia progresses rapidly, resulting in dyspnea, stridor, and cyanosis. The disease terminates with respiratory failure, and circulatory collapse.

Nonspecific laboratory findings include a leukocytosis, with a total WBC count up to 20,000 cells with increased bands, and greater than 80 percent polymorphonuclear cells. One also often finds increased fibrin split products in the blood indicative of a low-grade DIC. The BUN, creatinine, ALT, AST, and bilirubin may also be elevated, consistent with multiorgan failure.

In man, the mortality of untreated bubonic plague is approximately 60 percent (reduced to <5% with prompt effective therapy), whereas in untreated pneumonic plague the mortality rate is nearly 100 percent, and survival is unlikely if treatment is delayed beyond 18 hours of infection. In the U.S. in the past 50 years, 4 of the 7 pneumonic plague patients (57%) died. Recent data from the ongoing Madagascar epidemic, which began in 1989, corroborate that figure; the mortality associated with respiratory involvement was 57%, while that for bubonic plague was 15%.

DIAGNOSIS

Diagnosis is based primarily on clinical suspicion. The sudden appearance of large numbers of previously healthy patients with severe, rapidly progressive pneumonia with hemoptysis strongly suggests plague. A presumptive diagnosis can be made microscopically by identification of the coccobacillus in Gram, Wright, Giemsa, or Wayson's stained smears from lymph node needle aspirate, sputum, blood, or cerebrospinal fluid samples. When available, immunofluorescent staining is very useful. Definitive diagnosis relies on culturing the organism from blood, sputum, CSF, or bubo aspirates. The organism grows slowly at normal incubation temperatures, and may be misidentified by automated systems because of delayed biochemical reactions. It may be cultured on blood agar, MacConkey agar or infusion broth. Most naturally occurring strains of *Y. pestis* produce an F1-antigen *in vivo*, which can be detected in serum samples by immunoassay. A four-fold rise in antibody titer in patient serum is retrospectively diagnostic. PCR (using specific primers), although not sufficiently developed and evaluated for routine use, is a very sensitive and specific technique, currently able to identify as few as 10 organisms per ml. Most clinical assays can be performed in Biosafety Level 2 (BSL-2) labs, whereas procedures producing aerosols or yielding significant quantities of organisms require BSL-3 containment.

MEDICAL MANAGEMENT

Use Standard Precautions for bubonic plague patients. Suspected pneumonic plague cases require strict isolation with Droplet Precautions for at least 48 hours of antibiotic therapy, or until sputum cultures are negative in confirmed cases. If competent vectors (fleas) and reservoirs (rodents) are present, measures must be taken to prevent local disease cycles. These might include, but are not limited to, use of flea insecticides, rodent control measures (after or during flea control), and flea barriers for patient care areas.

Streptomycin, gentamicin, doxycycline, and chloramphenicol are highly effective, if begun early. Plague pneumonia is almost always fatal if treatment is not initiated within 24 hours of the onset of symptoms. Dosage regimens are as follows: streptomycin, 30 mg/kg/day IM in two divided doses; gentamicin, 5mg/kg IV once daily, or 2mg/kg loading dose followed by 1.75 mg/kg IV every 8 hours; doxycycline 200 mg initially, followed by 100 mg every 12 hours. Duration of therapy is 10 to 14 days. While the patient is typically afebrile after 3 days, the extra week of therapy prevents relapses. Results obtained from laboratory animal, but not human, experience, indicate that quinolone antibiotics, such as ciprofloxacin and ofloxacin, may also be effective. Recommended dosage of ciprofloxacin is 400mg IV twice daily. Chloramphenicol, 25 mg/kg IV loading dose followed by 15 mg/kg IV four times daily x 10-14 days, is required for the treatment of plague meningitis.

Usual supportive therapy includes IV crystalloids and hemodynamic monitoring. Although low-grade DIC may occur, clinically significant hemorrhage is uncommon, as is the need to treat with heparin. Endotoxic shock is common, but pressor agents are rarely needed. Finally, buboes rarely require any form of local care, but instead recede with systemic antibiotic therapy. In fact, incision and drainage poses a risk to others in contact with the patient; aspiration is recommended for diagnostic purposes and may provide symptomatic relief.

PROPHYLAXIS

Vaccine: No vaccine is currently available for prophylaxis of plague. A licensed, killed whole cell vaccine was available in the U.S. from 1946 until November 1998. It offered protection against bubonic plague, but was not effective against aerosolized *Y. pestis*. Presently, an F1-V antigen (fusion protein) vaccine is in development at USAMRIID. It protected mice for a year against an inhalational challenge, and is now being tested in primates.

Antibiotics: Face-to-face contacts (within 2 meters) of patients with pneumonic plague or persons possibly exposed to a plague aerosol in a plague BW attack) should be given antibiotic prophylaxis for seven days or the duration of risk of exposure plus seven days. If fever or cough occurs in these individuals, treatment with antibiotics should be started. Because of oral administration and relative lack of toxicity, the choice of antibiotic for prophylaxis is doxycycline 100 mg orally twice daily. Ciprofloxacin 500 mg orally twice daily has also shown to be effective in preventing disease in exposed mice, and may be more available in a wartime setting as it is also distributed in blister-packs for anthrax post-exposure prophylaxis. Tetracycline, 500mg orally four times daily, and chloramphenicol, 25 mg/kg orally four times daily, are acceptable alternatives. Contacts of bubonic plague patients need only be observed for symptoms for a week. If symptoms occur, start treatment antibiotics.

Q FEVER

SUMMARY

Signs and Symptoms: Fever, cough, and pleuritic chest pain may occur as early as ten days after exposure. Patients are not generally critically ill, and the illness lasts from 2 days to 2 weeks.

Diagnosis: Q fever is not a clinically distinct illness and may resemble a viral illness or other types of atypical pneumonia. The diagnosis is confirmed serologically.

Treatment: Q fever is generally a self-limited illness even without treatment, but tetracycline or doxycycline should be given orally for 5 to 7 days to prevent complications of the disease. Q fever endocarditis (rare) is much more difficult to treat.

Prophylaxis: Chemoprophylaxis begun too early during the incubation period may delay but not prevent the onset of symptoms. Therefore, tetracycline or doxycycline should be started 8-12 days post exposure and continued for 5 days. This regimen has been shown to prevent clinical disease. An inactivated whole cell IND vaccine is effective in eliciting protection against exposure, but severe local reactions to this vaccine may be seen in those who already possess immunity. Therefore, an intradermal skin test is recommended to detect pre-sensitized or immune individuals.

Isolation and Decontamination: Standard Precautions are recommended for healthcare workers. Person-to-person transmission is rare. Patients exposed to Q fever by aerosol do not present a risk for secondary contamination or re-aerosolization of the organism. Decontamination is accomplished with soap and water or a 0.5% chlorine solution on personnel. The M291 skin decontamination kit will not neutralize the organism.

OVERVIEW

The endemic form of Q fever is a zoonotic disease caused by the rickettsia, *Coxiella burnetii*. Its natural reservoirs are sheep, cattle, goats, dogs, cats and birds. The organism grows to especially high concentrations in placental tissues. The infected animals do not develop the disease, but do shed large numbers of the organisms in placental tissues and body fluids including milk, urine, and feces. Exposure to infected animals at parturition is an important risk factor for endemic disease. Humans acquire the disease by inhalation of aerosols contaminated with the organisms. Farmers and abattoir workers are at greatest risk occupationally. A biological warfare attack with Q fever would cause a disease similar to that occurring naturally. Q fever is also a significant hazard in laboratory personnel who are working with the organism.

HISTORY AND SIGNIFICANCE

Q fever was first described in Australia and called "Query fever" because the causative agent was initially unknown. *Coxiella burnetii*, discovered in 1937, is a rickettsial organism that is resistant to heat and desiccation and highly infectious by the aerosol route. A single inhaled organism may produce clinical illness. For all of these reasons, Q fever could be used by an adversary as an incapacitating biological warfare agent.

CLINICAL FEATURES

Following the usual incubation period of 2-14 days, Q fever generally occurs as a self-limiting febrile illness lasting 2 days to 2 weeks. The incubation period varies according to the numbers of organisms inhaled, with longer periods between exposure and illness with lower numbers of inhaled organisms (up to forty days in some cases). The disease generally presents as an acute non-differentiated febrile illness, with headaches, fatigue, and myalgias as prominent symptoms. Physical examination of the chest is usually normal. Pneumonia, manifested by an abnormal chest x-ray, occurs in half of all patients, but only around half of these, or 28 percent of patients, will have a cough (usually non-productive) or rales. Pleuritic chest pain occurs in about one-fourth of patients with Q fever pneumonia. Chest radiograph abnormalities, when present, are patchy infiltrates that may resemble viral or mycoplasma pneumonia. Rounded opacities and adenopathy have also been described.

Approximately 33 percent of Q fever cases will develop acute hepatitis. This can present with fever and abnormal liver function tests with the absence of pulmonary signs and symptoms. Uncommon complications include chronic hepatitis, culture-negative endocarditis, aseptic meningitis, encephalitis and osteomyelitis. Most patients who develop endocarditis have pre-existing valvular heart disease.

DIAGNOSIS

Differential Diagnosis: Since Q fever usually presents as an undifferentiated febrile illness, or a primary atypical pneumonia, it may be difficult to distinguish from viral illnesses and must be differentiated from pneumonia caused by *Mycoplasma pneumoniae, Legionella pneumophila, Chlamydia psittaci,* and *Chlamydia pneumoniae* (TWAR). More rapidly progressive forms of Q fever pneumonia may look like bacterial pneumonias such as tularemia or plague. Significant numbers of soldiers (from the same geographic area) presenting over a one to two week period with a nonspecific febrile illness, and associated pulmonary symptoms in about a quarter of cases, should trigger the treating physicians to consider the possibility of an attack with aerosolized Q fever. The diagnosis will often rest on the clinical and epidemiologic picture in the setting of a possible biowarfare attack.

Laboratory Diagnosis: A leukocytosis may be present in one third of patients. Most patients with Q fever have a mild elevation of hepatic transaminase levels. Identification of organisms by examination of the sputum is not helpful. Isolation of the organism is impractical, as the organism is difficult to culture and a significant hazard to laboratory workers. Serological tests for Q fever include identification of antibody to *C. burnetii* by indirect fluorescent antibody (IFA), enzyme-linked immunosorbent assay (ELISA), and complement fixation. Specific IgM antibodies may be detectable as early as the second week after onset of illness. ELISA testing is available at USAMRIID. A single serum specimen can be used to reliably diagnose acute Q fever with this test as early as 1 1/2 - 2 weeks into the illness. The most commonly available serologic test is the complement fixation test (CF) which is relatively insensitive and may not be useful if sera have intrinsic anti-complement activity.

MEDICAL MANAGEMENT

Standard Precautions are recommended for healthcare workers. Most cases of acute Q fever will eventually resolve without antibiotic treatment, but all suspected cases of Q fever should be treated to reduce the risk of complications. Tetracycline 500 mg every 6 hr or doxycycline 100 mg every 12 hr for 5-7 days will shorten the duration of illness, and fever usually disappears within one to two days after treatment is begun. Ciprofloxacin and other quinolones are active in vitro and should be considered in patients unable to take tetracycline or doxycycline. Successful treatment of Q fever endocarditis is much more difficult. Tetracycline or doxycycline given in combination with trimethoprim-sulfamethoxazolo (TMP-SMX) or rifampin for 12 months or longer has been successful in some cases. However, valve replacement is often required to achieve a cure.

PROPHYLAXIS

Vaccine: A formalin-inactivated whole cell IND vaccine is available for immunization of at-risk personnel on an investigational basis, although a Q fever vaccine is licensed in Australia. Vaccination with a single dose of this killed suspension of *C. burnetii* provides complete protection against naturally occurring Q fever, and greater than 95 percent protection against aerosol exposure. Protection lasts for at least 5 years. Administration of this vaccine in immune individuals may cause severe local induration, sterile abscess formation, and even necrosis at the inoculation site. This observation led to the development of an intradermal skin test using 0.02 mg of specific formalin-killed whole-cell vaccine to detect presensitized or immune individuals.

Antibiotics: Chemoprophylaxis using Tetracycline 500 mg every 6 hours or doxycycline 100 mg every 12 hours for 5–7 days is effective if begun 8-12 days post exposure. Chemoprophylaxis is not effective and may only prolong the onset of disease if given immediately (1 to 7 days) after exposure.

TULAREMIA

SUMMARY

Signs and Symptoms: Ulceroglandular tularemia presents with a local ulcer and regional lymphadenopathy, fever, chills, headache and malaise. Typhoidal tularemia presents with fever, headache, malaise, substernal discomfort, prostration, weight loss and a non-productive cough.

Diagnosis: Clinical diagnosis. Physical findings are usually non-specific. Chest x-ray may reveal a pneumonic process, mediastinal lymphadenopathy or pleural effusion. Routine culture is possible but difficult. The diagnosis can be established retrospectively by serology.

Treatment: Administration of antibiotics (streptomycin or gentamicin) with early treatment is very effective.

Prophylaxis: A live, attenuated vaccine is available as an investigational new drug. It is administered once by scarification. A two week course of tetracycline is effective as prophylaxis when given after exposure.

Isolation and Decontamination: Standard Precautions for healthcare workers. Organisms are relatively easy to render harmless by mild heat (55 degrees Celsius for 10 minutes) and standard disinfectants.

OVERVIEW

Francisella tularensis, the causative agent of tularemia, is a small, aerobic non-motile, gram-negative cocco-bacillus. Tularemia (also known as rabbit fever and deer fly fever) is a zoonotic disease that humans typically acquire after skin or mucous membrane contact with tissues or body fluids of infected animals, or from bites of infected ticks, deerflies, or mosquitoes. Less commonly, inhalation of contaminated dusts or ingestion of contaminated foods or water may produce clinical disease. Respiratory exposure by aerosol would typically cause typhoidal or pneumonic tularemia. *F. tularensis* can remain viable for weeks in water, soil, carcasses, hides, and for years in frozen rabbit meat. It is resistant for months to temperatures of freezing and below. It is easily killed by heat and disinfectants.

HISTORY AND SIGNIFICANCE

Tularemia was recognized in Japan in the early 1800's and in Russia in 1926. In the early 1900's, American workers investigating suspected plague epidemics in San Francisco isolated the organism and named it *Bacterium tularense* after Tulare County, California where the work was performed. Dr. Edward Francis, USPHS, established the cause of deer-fly fever as *Bacterium tularense* and subsequently devoted his life to researching the organism and disease, hence, the organism was later renamed *Francisella tularensis*

Francisella tularensis was weaponized by the United States in the 1950's and 1960's during the U.S.

offensive biowarfare program, and other countries are suspected to have weaponized this agent. This organism could potentially be stabilized for weaponization by an adversary and theoretically produced in either a wet or dried form, for delivery against U.S. forces in a similar fashion to the other bacteria discussed in this handbook.

CLINICAL FEATURES

After an incubation period varying from 1-21 days (average 3-5 days), presumably dependent upon the dose of organisms, onset is usually acute. Tularemia typically appears in one of six forms in man depending upon the route of inoculation: typhoidal, ulceroglandular, glandular, oculoglandular, oropharyngeal, and pneumonic tularemia. In humans, as few as 10 to 50 organisms will cause disease if inhaled or injected intradermally, whereas approximately 10^8 organisms are required with oral challenge.

Typhoidal tularemia (5-15 percent of naturally acquired cases) occurs mainly after inhalation of infectious aerosols, but can occur after intradermal or gastrointestinal challenge. *F. tularensis* would presumably be most likely delivered by aerosol in a BW attack and would primarily cause typhoidal tularemia. It manifests as fever, prostration, and weight loss, but unlike most other forms of the disease, presents without lymphadcnopathy. Pneumonia may be severe and fulminant and can be associated with any form of tularemia (30% of ulceroglandular cases), but it is most common in typhoidal tularemia (80% of cases). Respiratory symptoms, substernal discomfort, and a cough (productive and non-productive) may also be present. Case fatality rates following a BW attack may be greater than the 1-3 % seen with appropriately treated natural disease. Case fatality rates are about 35% in untreated naturally acquired typhoidal cases.

Ulceroglandular tularemia (75-85 percent of cases) is most often acquired through inoculation of the skin or mucous membranes with blood or tissue fluids of infected animals. It is characterized by fever, chills, headache, malaise, an ulcerated skin lesion, and painful regional lymphadenopathy. The skin lesion is usually located on the fingers or hand where contact occurs.

Glandular tularemia (5-10 percent of cases) results in fever and tender lymphadenopathy but no skin ulcer.

Oculoglandular tularemia (1-2 percent of cases) occurs after inoculation of the conjunctivae by contaminated hands, splattering of infected tissue fluids, or by aerosols. Patients have unilateral, painful, purulent conjunctivitis with preauricular or cervical lymphadenopathy. Chemosis, periorbital edema, and small nodular lesions or ulcerations of the palpebral conjunctiva are noted in some patients.

Oropharyngeal tularemia refers to primary ulceroglandular disease confined to the throat. It produces an acute exudative or membranous pharyngotonsillitis with cervical lymphadenopathy.

Pneumonic tularemia is a severe atypical pneumonia that may be fulminant and with a high case fatality rate if untreated. It can be primary following inhalation of organisms or • secondary following hematogenous / septicemic spread. It is seen in 30-80 percent of the typhoidal cases and in 10-15 percent of the ulceroglandular cases.

The case fatality rate without treatment is approximately 5 percent for the ulceroglandular form and 35 percent for the typhoidal form. All ages are susceptible, and recovery is generally followed by permanent immunity.

DIAGNOSIS

A clue to the diagnosis of tularemia subsequent to a BW attack with *F. tularensis* might be a large number of temporally clustered patients presenting with similar systemic illnesses and a non-productive pneumonia.

The clinical presentation of tularemia may be severe, yet non-specific. Differential diagnoses include typhoidal syndromes (e.g., salmonella, rickettsia, malaria) or pneumonic processes (e.g., plague, mycoplasma, SEB).

Radiologic evidence of pneumonia or mediastinal lymphadenopathy is most common with typhoidal disease. In general, chest radiographs show that approximately 50% of patients have pneumonia, and fewer than 1% have hilar adenopathy without parenchymal involvement. Pleural effusions are seen in 15% of patients with pneumonia. Interstitial patterns, cavitary lesions, bronchopleural fistulae, and calcifications have been reported in patients with tularemia pneumonia.

Laboratory diagnosis. Initial laboratory evaluations are generally nonspecific. Peripheral white blood cell count usually ranges from 5,000 to 22,000 cells per microliter. Differential blood cell counts are normal, with occasional lymphocytosis late in the disease. Hematocrit, hemoglobin, and platelet levels are usually normal. Mild elevations in lactic dehydrogenase, serum transaminases, and alkaline phosphatase are common. Rhabdomyolysis may be associated with elevations in serum creatine kinase and urinary myoglobin levels. Cerebrospinal fluid is usually normal, although mild abnormalities in protein, glucose, and blood cell count have been reported.

Tularemia can be diagnosed by recovery of the organism in culture from blood, ulcers, conjunctival exudates, sputum, gastric washings, and pharyngeal exudates. Recovery may even be possible after the institution of appropriate antibiotic therapy. The organism grows poorly on standard media but produces small, smooth, opaque colonies after 24 to 48 hours on media containing cysteine or other sulfhydryl compounds (e.g., glucose cysteine blood agar, thioglycollate broth). Isolation represents a clear hazard to laboratory personnel and culture should only be attempted in BSL-3 containment.

Most diagnoses of tularemia are made serologically using bacterial agglutination or enzyme-linked immunosorbent assay (ELISA). Antibodies to *F. tularensis* appear within the first week of infection but levels adequate to allow confidence in the specificity of the serologic diagnosis (titer > 1:160) do not appear until more than 2 weeks after infection. Because cross-reactions can occur with *Brucella* spp., Proteus OX19, and Yersinia organisms and because antibodies may persist for years after infection, diagnosis should be made only if a 4-fold or greater increase in the tularemia tube agglutination or microagglutination titer is seen during the course of the illness. Titers are usually negative the first week of infection, positive the second week in 50-70 percent of cases and reach a maximum in 4-8 weeks.

MEDICAL MANAGEMENT

Since there is no known human-to-human transmission, neither isolation nor quarantine are required, since Standard Precautions are appropriate for care of patients with draining lesions or pneumonia. Strict adherence to the drainage/secretion recommendations of Standard Precautions is required, especially for draining lesions, and for the disinfection of soiled clothing, bedding, equipment, etc. Heat and disinfectants easily inactivate the organism.

Appropriate therapy includes one of the following antibiotics:

- Gentamicin 3 - 5 mg/kg IV daily for 10 to 14 days
- Ciprofloxacin 400 mg IV every 12 hours, switch to oral ciprofloxacin (500 mg every 12 hours) after the

patient is clinically improved; continue for completion of a 10- to 14-day course of therapy

- Ciprofloxacin 750 mg orally every 12 hours for 10 to 14 days
- Streptomycin 7.5 - 10 mg/kg IM every 12 hours for 10 to 14 days

Streptomycin has historically been the drug of choice for tularemia; however, since it may not be readily available immediately after a large-scale BW attack, gentamicin and other alternative drugs should be considered first. Requests for streptomycin should be directed to the Roerig Streptomycin Program at Pfizer Pharmaceuticals in New York (800-254-4445). Another concern is that a fully virulent streptomycin-resistant strain of *F. tularensis* was developed during the 1950s and it is presumed that other countries have obtained it. The strain was sensitive to gentamicin. Gentamicin offers the advantage of providing broader coverage for gram-negative bacteria and may be useful when the diagnosis of tularemia is considered but in doubt.

In a recent study of treatment in 12 children with ulceroglandular tularemia, ciprofloxacin was satisfactory for outpatient treatment (Pediatric Infectious Disease Journal, 2000; 19:449-453). Tetracycline and chloramphenicol are also effective antibiotics;, however, they are associated with significant relapse rates.

PROPHYLAXIS

Vaccine: An investigational live-attenuated vaccine (Live Vaccine Strain - LVS), which is administered by scarification, has been given to >5,000 persons without significant adverse reactions and prevents typhoidal and ameliorates ulceroglandular forms of laboratory-acquired tularemia. Aerosol challenge tests in laboratory animals and human volunteers have demonstrated significant protection. As with all vaccines, the degree of protection depends upon the magnitude of the challenge dose. Vaccine-induced protection could be overwhelmed by extremely high doses of the tularemia bacteria.

Immunoprophylaxis. There is no passive immunoprophylaxis (i.e., immune globulin) available for pre- or post-exposure management of tularemia.

Pre-exposure prophylaxis: Chemoprophylaxis given for anthrax or plague (ciprofloxacin, doxycycline) may confer protection against tularemia, based on *in vitro* susceptibilities.

Post-exposure prophylaxis. A 2-week course of antibiotics is effective as post-exposure prophylaxis when given within 24 hours of aerosol exposure from a BW attack, using one of the following regimens:

- Ciprofloxacin 500 mg orally every 12 hours for 2 weeks
- Doxycycline 100 mg orally every 12 hours for 2 weeks
- Tetracycline 500 mg orally every 6 hours for 2 weeks

Chemoprophylaxis is not recommended following potential natural exposures (tick bite, rabbit or other animal exposures).

VIRAL AGENTS

Viruses are the simplest microorganisms and consist of a nucleocapsid protein coat containing genetic material, either RNA or DNA. In some cases, the viral particle is also surrounded by an outer lipid layer. Viruses are much smaller than bacteria and vary in size from 0.02 μm to 0.2 μm (1 μm = 1/1000 mm). Viruses are intracellular parasites and lack a system for their own metabolism; therefore, they are dependent on the synthetic machinery of their host cells. This means that viruses, unlike the bacteria, cannot be cultivated in synthetic nutritive solutions, but require living cells in order to multiply. The host cells can be from humans, animals, plants, or bacteria. Every virus requires its own special type of host cell for multiplication, because a complicated interaction occurs between the cell and virus. Virus-specific host cells can be cultivated in synthetic nutrient solutions and then infected with the virus in question. Another common way of cultivating viruses is to grow them on chorioallantoic membranes (from fertilized eggs). The cultivation of viruses is expensive, demanding, and time-consuming. A virus typically brings about changes in the host cell that eventually lead to cell death. This handbook covers three types of viruses which could potentially be employed as BW agents: smallpox, alphaviruses (eg., VEE), and hemorrhagic fever viruses.

SMALLPOX

SUMMARY

Signs and Symptoms: Clinical manifestations begin acutely with malaise, fever, rigors, vomiting, headache, and backache. 2-3 days later lesions appear which quickly progress from macules to papules, and eventually to pustular vesicles. They are more abundant on the extremities and face, and develop synchronously.

Diagnosis: Neither electron nor light microscopy are capable of discriminating variola from vaccinia, monkeypox or cowpox. The new PCR diagnostic techniques may be more accurate in discriminating between variola and other *Orthopoxviruses*.

Treatment: At present there is no effective chemotherapy, and treatment of a clinical case remains supportive.

Prophylaxis: Immediate vaccination or revaccination should be undertaken for all personnel exposed.

Isolation and Decontamination: Droplet and Airborne Precautions for a minimum of 17 days following exposure for all contacts. Patients should be considered infectious until all scabs separate and quarantined during this period. In the civilian setting strict quarantine of asymptomatic contacts may prove to be impractical and impossible to enforce. A reasonable alternative would be to require contacts to check their temperatures daily. Any fever above 38 C (101 F) during the 17-day period following exposure to a confirmed case would suggest the development of smallpox. The contact should then be isolated immediately, preferably at home, until smallpox is either confirmed or ruled out and remain in isolation until all scabs separate.

OVERVIEW

Smallpox is caused by the Orthopox virus, variola, which occurs in at least two strains, variola major and the milder disease, variola minor. Despite the global eradication of smallpox and continued availability of a vaccine, the potential weaponization of variola continues to pose a military threat. This threat can be attributed to the aerosol infectivity of the virus, the relative ease of large-scale production, and an increasingly *Orthopoxvirus*-naive populace. Although the fully developed cutaneous eruption of smallpox is unique, earlier stages of the rash could be mistaken for varicella. Secondary spread of infection constitutes a nosocomial hazard from the time of onset of a smallpox patient's exanthem until scabs have separated. Quarantine with respiratory isolation should be applied to secondary contacts for 17 days post-exposure. Vaccinia vaccination and vaccinia immune globulin each possess some efficacy in post-exposure prophylaxis.

HISTORY AND SIGNIFICANCE

Endemic smallpox was declared eradicated in 1980 by the World Health Organization (WHO). Although two WHO-approved repositories of variola virus remain at the Centers for Disease Control and Prevention (CDC) in Atlanta and the Institute for Viral Preparations in Moscow, the extent of clandestine stockpiles in other parts of the world remains unknown. In January 1996, WHO's governing board recommended that all stocks of smallpox be destroyed by 30 June 1999. However, action on this was delayed by the Clinton administration in May 1999 due to concerns over the need for further study of the virus given its potential as a biological warfare agent. The smallpox stockpiles are now scheduled for destruction on 30 June 2002.

The United States stopped vaccinating its military population in 1989 and civilians in the early 1980s. These populations are now susceptible to variola major, although recruits immunized in 1989 may retain some degree of immunity. Variola may have been used by the British Army against native Americans by giving them contaminated blankets from the beds of smallpox victims during the eighteenth century. Japan considered the use of smallpox as a BW weapon in World War II and it has been considered as a possible threat agent against US forces for many years. In addition, the former Soviet Union is reported to have produced and stockpiled massive quantities of the virus for use as a biological weapon. It is not known whether these stockpiles still exist in Russia.

CLINICAL FEATURES

The incubation period of smallpox averaged 12 days, although it could range from 7-19 days following exposure. Clinical manifestations begin acutely with malaise, fever, rigors, vomiting, headache, and backache; 15% of patients developed delirium. Approximately 10% of light-skinned patients exhibited an erythematous rash during this phase. Two to three days later, an enanthem appears concomitantly with a discrete rash about the face, hands and forearms.

Following eruptions on the lower extremities, the rash spread centrally to the trunk over the next week. Lesions quickly progressed from macules to papules, and eventually to pustular vesicles. Lesions were more abundant on the extremities and face, and this centrifugal distribution is an important diagnostic feature. In distinct contrast to varicella, lesions on various segments of the body remain generally synchronous in their stages of development. From 8 to 14 days after onset, the pustules form scabs that leave depressed depigmented scars upon healing. Although variola concentrations in the throat, conjunctiva, and urine diminish with time, virus can be readily recovered from scabs throughout convalescence. Therefore, patients should be isolated and considered infectious until all scabs separate.

For the past century, two distinct types of smallpox were recognized. Variola minor was distinguished by milder systemic toxicity and more diminutive pox lesions, and caused 1% mortality in unvaccinated victims. However, the prototypical disease variola major caused mortality of 3% and 30% in the vaccinated and unvaccinated, respectively. Other clinical forms associated with variola major, flat-type and hemorrhagic type smallpox were notable for severe mortality. A naturally occurring relative of variola, monkeypox, occurs in Africa, and is clinically indistinguishable from smallpox with the exception of a lower case fatality rate and notable enlargement of cervical and inguinal lymph nodes.

DIAGNOSIS

Smallpox must be distinguished from other vesicular exanthems, such as chickenpox, erythema multiforme with bullae, or allergic contact dermatitis. Particularly problematic to infection control measures would be the failure to recognize relatively mild cases of smallpox in persons with partial immunity. An additional threat to effective quarantine is the fact that exposed persons may shed virus from the oropharynx without ever manifesting disease. Therefore, quarantine and initiation of medical countermeasures should be promptly followed by an accurate diagnosis so as to avert panic.

The usual method of diagnosis is demonstration of characteristic virions on electron microscopy of vesicular scrapings. Under light microscopy, aggregations of variola virus particles, called Guarnieri bodies are found. Another rapid but relatively insensitive test for Guarnieri bodies in vesicular scrapings is Gispen's modified silver stain, in which cytoplasmic inclusions appear black.

None of the above laboratory tests are capable of discriminating variola from vaccinia, monkeypox or cowpox. This differentiation classically required isolation of the virus and characterization of its growth on chorioallantoic membrane. The development of polymerase chain reaction diagnostic techniques promises a more accurate and less cumbersome method of discriminating between variola and other *Orthopoxviruses*.

MEDICAL MANAGEMENT

Medical personnel must be prepared to recognize a vesicular exanthem in possible biowarfare theaters as potentially variola, and to initiate appropriate countermeasures. Any confirmed case of smallpox should be considered an international emergency with immediate report made to public health authorities. Droplet and Airborne Precautions for a minimum of 17 days following exposure for *all* persons in direct contact with the index case, especially the unvaccinated. In the civilian setting strict quarantine of asymptomatic contacts may prove to be impractical and impossible to enforce. A reasonable alternative would be to require contacts to check their temperatures daily. Any fever above 38 C (101 F) during the 17-day period following exposure to a confirmed case would suggest the development of smallpox. The contact should then be isolated immediately, preferably at home, until smallpox is either confirmed or ruled out and remain in isolation until all scabs separate. Patients should be considered infectious until all scabs separate. Immediate vaccination or revaccination should also be undertaken for all personnel exposed to either weaponized variola virus or a clinical case of smallpox.

The potential for airborne spread to other than close contacts is controversial. In general, close person-to-person contact Is required for transmission to reliably occur. Nevertheless, variola's potential in low relative humidity for airborne dissemination was alarming in two hospital outbreaks. Smallpox patients were infectious from the time of onset of their eruptive exanthem, most commonly from days 3-6 after onset of fever. Infectivity was markedly enhanced if the patient manifested a cough. Indirect transmission via contaminated bedding or other fomites was infrequent. Some close contacts harbored virus in their throats without developing disease, and hence might have served as a means of secondary transmission.

Vaccination with a verified clinical "take" (vesicle with scar formation) within the past 3 years is considered to render a person immune to smallpox. However, given the difficulties and uncertainties under wartime conditions of verifying the adequacy of troops' prior vaccination, routine revaccination of all potentially exposed personnel would seem prudent if there existed a significant prospect of smallpox exposure.

Antivirals for use against smallpox are under investigation. Cidofovir has been shown to have significant *in vitro* and *in vivo* activity in experimental animals. Whether it would offer benefit superior to immediate post-exposure vaccination in humans has not been determined.

PROPHYLAXIS

Vaccine: Smallpox vaccine (vaccinia virus) is most often administered by intradermal inoculation with a bifurcated needle, a process that became known as scarification because of the permanent scar that resulted. Vaccination after exposure to weaponized smallpox or a case of smallpox may prevent or ameliorate disease if given as soon as possible and preferably within 7 days after exposure. A vesicle typically appears at the vaccination site 5-7 days post-inoculation, with surrounding erythema and induration. The lesion forms a scab and gradually heals over the next 1-2 weeks.

Side effects include low-grade fever and axillary lymphadenopathy. The attendant erythema and induration of the vaccination vesicle is frequently misdiagnosed as bacterial superinfection. More severe first-time vaccine reactions include secondary inoculation of the virus to other sites such as the face, eyelid, or other persons (~ 6/10,000 vaccinations), and generalized vaccinia, which is a systemic spread of the virus to produce mucocutaneous lesions away from the primary vaccination site (~3/10,000 vaccinations).

Vaccination is *contraindicated* in the following conditions: immunosuppression, HIV infection, history or evidence of eczema, or current household, sexual, or other close physical contact with person(s) possessing one of these conditions. In addition, vaccination should not be performed during pregnancy. Despite these caveats, most authorities state that, with the exception of significant impairment of systemic immunity, there are no absolute contraindications to *post-exposure* vaccination of a person who experiences *bona fide* exposure to variola. However, concomitant VIG administration is recommended for pregnant and eczematous persons in such circumstances.

Passive Immunoprophylaxis: Vaccinia Immune Globulin (VIG) is generally indicated for treatment of complications to the smallpox (vaccinia) vaccine, and should be available when administering vaccine. Limited data suggests that vaccinia immune globulin may be of value in post-exposure prophylaxis of smallpox when given within the first week following exposure, and concurrently with vaccination. Vaccination alone is recommended for those without contraindications to the vaccine. If greater than one week has elapsed after exposure, administration of both products, if available, is reasonable. The dose for prophylaxis or treatment is 0.6 ml/kg intramuscularly. Due to the large volume (42 mls in a 70 Kg person), the dose would be given in multiple sites over 24-36 hours.

VENEZUELAN EQUINE ENCEPHALITIS

SUMMARY

Signs and Symptoms: Incubation period 1-6 days. Acute systemic febrile illness with encephalitis developing in a small percentage (4% children; < 1% adults). Generalized malaise, spiking fevers, rigors, severe headache, photophobia, and myalgias for 24-72 hours. Nausea, vomiting, cough, sore throat, and diarrhea may follow. Full recovery from malaise and fatigue takes 1-2 weeks. The incidence of CNS disease and associated morbidity and mortality would be much higher after a BW attack.

Diagnosis: Clinical and epidemiological diagnosis. Physical findings non-specific. The white blood cell count may show a striking leukopenia and lymphopenia. Virus isolation may be made from serum, and in some cases throat swab specimens. Both neutralizing or IgG antibody in paired sera or VEE specific IgM present in a single serum sample indicate recent infection.

Therapy: Treatment is supportive only. Treat uncomplicated VEE infections with analgesics to relieve headache and myalgia. Patients who develop encephalitis may require anticonvulsants and intensive supportive care to maintain fluid and electrolyte balance, ensure adequate ventilation, and avoid complicating secondary bacterial infections.

Prophylaxis: A live, attenuated vaccine is available as an investigational new drug. A second, formalin-inactivated, killed vaccine is available for boosting antibody titers in those initially receiving the first vaccine. No post-exposure immunoprophylaxis. In experimental animals, alpha-interferon and the interferon-inducer poly-ICLC have proven highly effective as post-exposure prophylaxis. There are no human clinical data.

Isolation and Decontamination: Patient isolation and quarantine is not required. Standard Precautions augmented with vector control while the patient is febrile. There is no evidence of direct human-to-human or horse-to-human transmission. The virus can be destroyed by heat (80°C for 30 min) and standard disinfectants.

OVERVIEW

The Venezuelan equine encephalitis (VEE) virus complex is a group of eight mosquito-borne alphaviruses that are endemic in northern South America and Trinidad and causes rare cases of human encephalitis in Central America, Mexico, and Florida. These viruses can cause severe diseases in humans and Equidae (horses, mules, burros and donkeys). Natural infections are acquired by the bites of a wide variety of mosquitoes. Equidae serve as amplifying hosts and source of mosquito infection.

Western and Eastern Equine Encephalitis viruses are similar to the VEE complex, are often difficult to distinguish clinically, and share similar aspects of transmission and epidemiology. The human infective dose for VEE is considered to be 10-100 organisms, which is one of the principal reasons that VEE is considered a militarily effective BW agent. Neither the population density of infected mosquitoes nor the aerosol concentration of virus particles has to be great to allow significant transmission of VEE in a BW attack. There is no evidence of direct human-to-human or horse-to-human transmission. Natural aerosol transmission is not known to occur. VEE particles are not considered stable in the environment, and are thus not as persistent as the bacteria responsible for Q fever, tularemia or anthrax. Heat and standard disinfectants can easily kill the VEE virus complex.

HISTORY AND SIGNIFICANCE

Between 1969 and 1971, an epizootic of a "highly pathogenic strain" of VEE emerged in Guatemala, moved through Mexico, and entered Texas in June 1971. This strain was virulent in both equine species and humans. In Mexico, there were 8,000-10,000 equine deaths, "tens of thousands" of equine cases, and 17,000 human cases (no human deaths). Over 10,000 horses in Texas died. Once the Texas border was breached, a national emergency was declared and resources were mobilized to vaccinate equines in 20 states (95% of all horses and donkeys were vaccinated; over 3.2 million animals), establish equine quarantines, and control mosquito populations with broad-scale insecticide use in the Rio Grande Valley and along the Gulf Coast. A second VEE outbreak in 1995 in Venezuela and Columbia involved over 75,000 human cases and over 20 deaths.

VEE is better characterized than EEE or WEE, primarily because it was tested as a BW agent during the U.S. offensive program in the 1950's and 1960's. Other countries have also been or are suspected to have weaponized this agent. In compliance with President Nixon's National Security Decision No. 35 of November 1969 to destroy the BW microbial stockpile, all existing stocks of VEE in the U.S. were publicly destroyed.

These viruses could theoretically be produced in large amounts in either a wet or dried form by relatively unsophisticated and inexpensive systems. This form of the VEE virus complex could be intentionally disseminated as an aerosol and would be highly infectious. It could also be spread by the purposeful dissemination of infected mosquitoes, which can probably transmit the virus throughout their lives. The VEE complex is relatively stable during the storage and manipulation procedures necessary for weaponization.

In natural human epidemics, severe and often fatal encephalitis in Equidae (30-90% mortality) always precedes disease in humans. However, a biological warfare attack with virus intentionally disseminated as an aerosol would most likely cause human disease as a primary event or simultaneously with Equidae. During natural epidemics, illness or death in wild or free ranging Equidae may not be recognized before the onset of human disease, thus a natural epidemic could be confused with a BW event, and data on onset of disease should be considered with caution. A more reliable method for determining the likelihood of a BW event would be the presence of VEE outside of its natural geographic range. A biological warfare attack in a region populated by Equidae and appropriate mosquito vectors could initiate an epizootic/epidemic.

CLINICAL FEATURES

Susceptibility is high (90-100%), and nearly 100% of those infected develop overt illnesses. The overall case fatality rate for VEE is < 1%, although it is somewhat higher in the very young or aged. Recovery from an infection results in excellent short-term and long-term immunity.

93

VEE is primarily an acute, incapacitating, febrile illness with encephalitis developing in only a small percentage of the infected population. Most VEE infections are mild (EEE and WEE are predominantly encephalitis infections). After an incubation period from 1-6 days, onset is usually sudden. The acute phase lasts 24-72 hours and is manifested by generalized malaise, chills, spiking high fevers (38°C-40.5°C), rigors, severe headache, photophobia, and myalgias in the legs and lumbosacral area. Nausea, vomiting, cough, sore throat, and diarrhea may follow. Physical signs include conjunctival injection, erythematous pharynx and muscle tenderness. Patients would be incapacitated by malaise and fatigue for 1-2 weeks before full recovery.

During natural epidemics, approximately 4% of infected children (<15 years old) and less than 1% of adults will develop signs of severe CNS infection (35% fatality for children and 10% for adults). Adults rarely develop neurologic complications during natural infections. Experimental aerosol challenges in animals suggest that the incidence of CNS disease and associated morbidity and mortality would be much higher after a BW attack, as the VEE virus would infect the olfactory nerve and spread directly to the CNS. Mild CNS findings would include lethargy, somnolence, or mild confusion, with or without nuchal rigidity. Seizures, ataxia, paralysis, or coma follow more severe CNS involvement. VEE infection during pregnancy may cause encephalitis in the fetus, placental damage, abortion, or severe congenital neuroanatomical anomalies.

DIAGNOSIS

Diagnosis of VEE is suspected on clinical and epidemiological grounds, but confirmed by virus isolation, serology and PCR. A variety of serological tests are applicable, including the IgM ELISA indirect FA, hemagglutination inhibition, complement-fixation, and IgG. For persons without prior known exposure to VEE complex viruses, a presumptive diagnosis may be made by identifying IgM antibody in a single serum sample taken 5-7 days after onset of illness. PCR procedures are available for confirmation, but are generally available only as a rear laboratory capability.

Samples suitable for performing diagnostic tests include blood culture (only in appropriate BSL-3 containment), acute and convalescent sera, and cerebrospinal fluid. Viremia during the acute phase of the illness (but not during encephalitis) is generally high enough to allow detection by antigen-capture enzyme-linked immunosorbent assay (ELISA). Virus isolation is time consuming, but can be performed from serum and throat swab specimens by inoculation of cell cultures or suckling mice (a Gold Standard identification assay for VEE). VEE should be isolated only in a BSL-3 laboratory.

The white blood cell count shows a striking leukopenia and lymphopenia. In cases with encephalitis, the cerebrospinal fluid pressure may be increased and contain up to 1,000 WBCs/mm^3 (predominantly mononuclear cells) and a mildly elevated protein concentration.

An outbreak of VEE may be difficult to distinguish from influenza on clinical grounds. Clues to the diagnosis are the appearance of a small proportion of neurological cases, or disease in equine animals. However, these indicators may be absent in a BW attack. A BW aerosol attack could lead to an epidemic of febrile meningoencephalitis featuring seizures and coma. In a BW context, the differential diagnosis would include other causes of aseptic meningitis and meningoencephalitis.

MEDICAL MANAGEMENT

No specific viral therapy exists; hence treatment is supportive only. Patients with uncomplicated VEE infection may be treated with analgesics to relieve headache and myalgia. Patients who develop encephalitis may require anticonvulsants and intensive supportive care to maintain fluid and electrolyte balance, ensure adequate ventilation, and avoid complicating secondary bacterial infections. Patients should be treated in a screened room or in quarters treated with a residual insecticide for at least 5 days after onset, or until afebrile, as human cases may be infectious for mosquitoes for at least 72 hours. Patient isolation and quarantine is not required; sufficient contagion control is provided by the implementation of Standard Precautions augmented with the need for vector control while the patient is febrile. Patient-to-patient transmission by means of respiratory droplet infection has not been proven. The virus can be destroyed by heat (80 C for 30 min) and standard disinfectants.

PROPHYLAXIS

Vaccine: There are two IND human unlicensed VEE vaccines. The first investigational vaccine (designated TC-83) was developed in the 1960's and is a live, attenuated cell-culture-propagated vaccine produced by the Salk Institute. This vaccine is not effective against all of the serotypes in the VEE complex. It has been used to protect several thousand persons against laboratory infections and is presently licensed for use in Equidae (and was used in the 1970-71 Texas epizootic in horses), but is an IND vaccine for humans. The vaccine is given as a single 0.5 mL subcutaneous dose. Fever, malaise, and headache occur in approximately 20 percent of vaccinees, and may be moderate to severe in 10 percent of those vaccinees to warrant bed rest for 1-2 days. Another 18 percent of vaccinees fail to develop detectable neutralizing antibodies, but it is unknown whether they are susceptible to clinical infection if challenged. Temporary contraindications for use include a concurrent viral infection or pregnancy.

A second investigational (IND) vaccine (designated C-84) has been tested but not licensed in humans and is prepared by formalin-inactivation of the TC-83 strain. This vaccine is not used for primary immunization, but is used to boost nonresponders to TC-83. Administer 0.5 mL subcutaneously at 2-4 week intervals for up to 3 inoculations or until an antibody response is measured. Periodic boosters are required. The C-84 vaccine alone does not protect rodents against experimental aerosol challenge. Therefore, C-83 is used only as a booster immunogen for the TC-84 vaccine.

As with all vaccines, the degree of protection depends upon the magnitude of the challenge dose; vaccine-induced protection could be overwhelmed by extremely high doses of the pathogen. Research is underway to produce a recombinant VEE vaccine.

Immunoprophylaxis: At present, there is no pre-exposure or post-exposure immunoprophylaxis available.

Chemoprophylaxis: In experimental animals, alpha-interferon and the interferon-inducer poly-ICLC have proven highly effective for post-exposure chemoprophylaxis of VEE. There are no clinical data on which to assess efficacy of these drugs in humans.

VIRAL HEMORRHAGIC FEVERS

SUMMARY

Signs and Symptoms: VHFs are febrile illnesses which can feature flushing of the face and chest, petechiae, bleeding, edema, hypotension, and shock. Malaise, myalgias, headache, vomiting, and diarrhea may occur in any of the hemorrhagic fevers.

Diagnosis: Definitive diagnosis rests on specific virologic techniques. Significant numbers of military personnel with a hemorrhagic fever syndrome should suggest the diagnosis of a viral hemorrhagic fever.

Treatment: Intensive supportive care may be required. Antiviral therapy with ribavirin may be useful in several of these infections (Available only as IND under protocol). Convalescent plasma may be effective in Argentine hemorrhagic fever (Available only as IND under protocol).

Prophylaxis: The only licensed VHF vaccine is yellow fever vaccine. Prophylactic ribavirin may be effective for Lassa fever, Rift Valley fever, CCHF, and possibly HFRS (Available only as IND under protocol).

Isolation and Decontamination: Contact isolation, with the addition of a surgical mask and eye protection for those coming within three feet of the patient, is indicated for suspected or proven Lassa fever, CCHF, or filovirus infections. Respiratory protection should be upgraded to airborne isolation, including the use of a fit-tested HEPA filtered respirator, a battery powered air purifying respirator, or a positive pressure supplied air respirator, if patients with the above conditions have prominent cough, vomiting, diarrhea, or hemorrhage. Decontamination is accomplished with hypochlorite or phenolic disinfectants.

OVERVIEW

The viral hemorrhagic fevers are a diverse group of illnesses caused by RNA viruses from four viral families. The *Arenaviridae* include the etiologic agents of Argentine, Bolivian, and Venezuelan hemorrhagic fevers, and Lassa fever. The *Bunyaviridae* include the members of the *Hantavirus* genus, the Congo-Crimean hemorrhagic fever virus from the *Nairovirus* genus, and the Rift Valley fever virus from the *Phlebovirus* genus; the *Filoviridae* include Ebola and Marburg viruses; and the *Flaviviridae* include dengue and yellow fever viruses. These viruses are spread in a variety of ways; some may be transmitted to humans through a respiratory portal of entry. Although evidence for weaponization does not exist for many of these viruses, they are included in this handbook because of their *potential* for aerosol dissemination or weaponization, or likelihood for confusion with similar agents that might be weaponized.

HISTORY AND SIGNIFICANCE

Because these viruses are so diverse and occur in different geographic locations endemically, their full history is beyond the scope of this handbook. However, there are some significant events that may provide insight into their possible importance as biological threat agents.

Arenaviridae: Argentine hemorrhagic fever (AHF), caused by the Junin virus, was first described in 1955 in corn harvesters. From 300 to 600 cases per year occur in areas of the Argentine pampas. Bolivian,

Brazilian, and Venezuelan hemorrhagic fevers are caused by the related Machupo, Guanarito, and Sabia viruses. Lassa virus causes disease in West Africa. These viruses are transmitted from their rodent reservoirs to humans by the inhalation of dusts contaminated with rodent excreta.

Bunyaviridae: Congo-Crimean hemorrhagic fever (CCHF) is a tick-borne disease that occurs in the Crimea and in parts of Africa, Europe and Asia. It can also be spread by contact with infected animals, and in healthcare settings. Rift Valley fever (RVF) is a mosquito-borne disease that occurs in Africa. The hantaviruses are rodent-borne viruses with a wide geographic distribution. Hantaan and closely related viruses cause hemorrhagic fever with renal syndrome (HFRS), (also known as Korean hemorrhagic fever or epidemic hemorrhagic fever). This is the most common disease due to hantaviruses. It was described prior to WW II in Manchuria along the Amur River, among United Nations troops during the Korean conflict, and subsequently in Japan, China, and in the Russian Far East. Severe disease also occurs in some Balkan states, including Bosnia, Serbia and Greece. Nephropathia epidemica is a milder disease that occurs in Scandinavia and other parts of Europe, and is caused by strains carried by bank voles. In addition, newly described hantaviruses cause Hantavirus Pulmonary Syndrome (HPS) in the Americas. The hantaviruses are transmitted to humans by the inhalation of dusts contaminated with rodent excreta.

Filoviridae: Ebola hemorrhagic fever was first recognized in the western equatorial province of the Sudan and the nearby region of Zaire in 1976. A second outbreak occurred in Sudan in 1979, and in 1995 a large outbreak (316 cases) developed in Kikwit, Zaire, from a single index case. Subsequent epidemics have occurred in Gabon and the Ivory Coast. The African strains cause severe disease and death. It is not known why this disease appears infrequently. A related virus (Ebola Reston) was isolated from monkeys imported into the United States from the Philippines in 1989, and subsequently developed hemorrhagic fever. While subclinical infections occurred among exposed animal handlers, Ebola Reston has not been identified as a human pathogen. Marburg epidemics have occurred on six occasions: five times in Africa, and once in Europe. The first recognized outbreak occurred in Marburg, Germany, and Yugoslavia, among people exposed to African green monkeys, and resulted in 31 cases and 7 deaths. Filoviruses can be spread from human to human by direct contact with infected blood, secretions, organs, or semen. Ebola Reston apparently spread from monkey to monkey, and from monkeys to humans by the respiratory route. The natural reservoirs of the filoviruses are unknown.

Flaviviridae: Yellow fever and dengue are two mosquito-borne fevers that have great importance in the history of military campaigns and military medicine. Tick-borne flaviviruses include the agents of Kyanasur Forest disease in India, and Omsk hemorrhagic fever in Siberia.

All of the VHF agents (except for dengue virus) are infectious by aerosol in the laboratory. These viruses could conceivably be used by an adversary as biological warfare agents, in view of their aerosol infectivity, and, for some viruses, high lethality.

CLINICAL FEATURES

The clinical syndrome that these viruses may cause is generally referred to as viral hemorrhagic fever, or VHF. The target organ in the VHF syndrome is the vascular bed; accordingly, the dominant clinical features are usually due to microvascular damage and changes in vascular permeability.

Not all infected patients develop VHF. There is both divergence and uncertainty about which host factors and viral strain characteristics might be responsible for the mechanisms of disease. For example, an immunopathogenic mechanism has been identified for dengue hemorrhagic fever, which usually occurs among patients previously infected with a heterologous dengue serotype. Antibody directed against the previous strain enhances uptake of dengue virus by circulating monocytes. These cells express viral antigens on their surfaces. Lysis of the infected monocytes by cytotoxic T-cell responses results in the release of pro-inflammatory cytokines, pro-coagulants, and anticoagulants, which in turn results in vascular injury and permeability, complement activation, and a systemic coagulopathy.

DIC has been implicated in Rift Valley, Marburg and Ebola fevers, but in most VHFs the etiology of the coagulopathy is multifactorial (e.g., hepatic damage, consumptive coagulopathy, and primary marrow injury to megakaryocytes).

Common symptoms are fever, myalgia, and prostration. Physical examination may reveal only conjunctival injection, mild hypotension, flushing, and petechial hemorrhages. Full-blown VHF typically evolves to shock and generalized mucous membrane hemorrhage, and often is accompanied by evidence of pulmonary hematopoietic, and neurologic involvement. Renal insufficiency is proportional to cardiovascular compromise, except in HFRS, which features renal failure as an integral part of the disease process.

Apart from epidemiologic and intelligence information, some distinctive clinical features may suggest a specific etiologic agent. While hepatic involvement is common among the VHFs, a clinical picture dominated by jaundice and other features of hepatitis is only seen in some cases of Rift Valley fever, Congo-Crimean, Marburg, and Ebola HFs, and yellow fever. Kyanasur Forest disease and Omsk hemorrhagic fever are notable for pulmonary involvement, and a biphasic illness with subsequent CNS manifestations. Among the arenavirus infections, Lassa fever can cause severe peripheral edema due to capillary leak, but hemorrhage is uncommon, while hemorrhage Is commonly caused by the South American arenaviruses. Severe hemorrhage and nosocomial transmission are typical for Congo-Crimean HF. Retinitis is commonly seen in Rift Valley fever, and hearing loss is common among Lassa fever survivors.

Because of their worldwide occurrence, additional consideration should be given to hantavirus infections. Classic HFRS has a severe course that progresses sequentially from fever through hemorrhage, shock, renal failure, and polyuria. Nephropathia endemica features prominent fever, myalgia, abdominal pain, and oliguria, without shock or severe hemorrhagic manifestations. North American cases of Hantavirus Pulmonary Syndrome (HPS) due to the Sin Nombre virus lack hemorrhagic manifestations and renal failure, but nevertheless carry a very high mortality due to rapidly progressive and severe pulmonary capillary leak, which presents as ARDS. These syndromes may overlap. Subclinical or clinical pulmonary edema may occur in HFRS and nephropathica endemica, while HFRS has complicated HPS due to South American hantaviruses and the Bayou and Black Creek Canal viruses in North America.

Mortality may be substantial, ranging from 0.2% percent for nephropathia endemica, to 50 to 90 percent among Ebola victims.

DIAGNOSIS

A detailed travel history and a high index of suspicion are essential in making the diagnosis of VHF. Patients with arenavirus or hantavirus infections often recall having seen rodents during the presumed incubation period, but since the viruses are spread to man by aerosolized excreta or environmental contamination, actual contact with the reservoir is not necessary. Large mosquito populations are common during Rift Valley fever or flavivirus transmission, but a history of mosquito bite is too common to be of diagnostic importance, whereas tick bites or nosocomial exposure are of some significance in suspecting Congo-Crimean HF. Large numbers of military personnel presenting with VHF manifestations in the same geographic area over a short time period should lead treating medical care providers to suspect either a natural outbreak in an endemic setting, or possibly a biowarfare attack, particularly if this type of disease does not occur naturally in the local area.

VHF should be suspected in any patient presenting with a severe febrile illness and evidence of vascular involvement (postural hypotension, petechiae, easy bleeding, flushing of face and chest, non-dependent edema) who has traveled to an area where the virus is known to occur, or where intelligence information suggests a biological warfare threat. Symptoms and signs suggesting additional organ system involvement are common (headache, photophobia, pharyngitis, cough, nausea or vomiting, diarrhea, constipation, abdominal pain, hyperesthesia, dizziness, confusion, tremor), but usually do not dominate the picture with the exceptions listed above under "Clinical Features." A positive tourniquet test has been particularly useful in dengue hemorrhagic fever, but should be sought in other hemorrhagic fevers as well.

The clinical laboratory can be very helpful. Thrombocytopenia (exception: Lassa) and leukopenia (exceptions: Lassa, Hantaan, and some severe CCHF cases) are the rule. Proteinuria and/or hematuria are common, and their presence is the rule for Argentine HF, Bolivian HF, and HFRS. High AST elevation correlates with severity of Lassa fever, and jaundice is a poor prognostic sign in yellow fever.

In most geographic areas, the major item in the differential diagnosis is malaria. It must be borne in mind that parasitemia in patients partially immune to malaria does not prove that symptoms are due to malaria. Other items in the differential may include typhoid fever, nontyphoidal salmonellosis, leptospirosis, rickettsial infections, shigellosis, relapsing fever, fulminant hepatitis, and meningococcemia. Additional illnesses which could mimic VHF include acute leukemia, lupus erythematosus, idiopathic or thrombotic thrombocytopenic purpura, hemolytic uremic syndrome and the multiple causes of disseminated intravascular coagulation.

Definitive diagnosis in an individual case rests on specific virologic diagnosis. Most patients have readily detectable viremia at presentation (exception: hantaviral infections). Rapid enzyme immunoassays can detect viral antigens in acute sera from patients with Argentine HF, Lassa fever, Rift Valley fever, Congo-Crimean HF, and yellow fever. Lassa- and Hantaan-specific IgM often are detectable during the acute illness. Diagnosis by virus cultivation and identification will require 3 to 10 days or longer. With the exception of dengue, specialized microbiologic containment is required for safe handling of these viruses. Appropriate precautions should be observed in collection, handling, shipping, and processing of diagnostic samples. Both the Centers for Disease Control and Prevention (CDC, Atlanta, Georgia) and the U.S. Army Medical Research Institute of Infectious Diseases (USAMRIID, Frederick, Maryland) have diagnostic laboratories functioning at the highest (BL-4 or P-4) containment level.

MEDICAL MANAGEMENT

General principles of supportive care apply to hemodynamic, hematologic, pulmonary, and neurologic manifestations of VHF, regardless of the specific etiologic agent. Only intensive care will save the most severely ill patients. Health care providers employing vigorous fluid resuscitation of hypotensive patients must be mindful of the propensity of some VHFs (e.g., HFRS) for pulmonary capillary leak. Pressor agents are frequently required. The use of intravascular devices and invasive hemodynamic monitoring must be carefully considered in the context of potential benefit versus the risk of hemorrhage. Restlessness, confusion, myalgia, and hyperesthesia should be managed by conservative measures, and the judicious use of sedatives and analgesics. Secondary infections may occur as with any patient undergoing intensive care utilizing invasive proceduroc and devices, such as intravenous lines and indwelling catheters.

The management of clinical bleeding should follow the same principles as for any patient with a systemic coagulopathy, assisted by coagulation studies. Intramuscular injections, aspirin and other anticoagulant drugs should be avoided.

The investigational antiviral drug ribavirin is available via compassionate use protocols for therapy of Lassa fever, HFRS, Congo-Crimean HF, and Rift Valley fever. Separate Phase III efficacy trials have indicated that parenteral ribavirin reduces morbidity in HFRS, and lowers both the morbidity and mortality of Lassa fever. In the HFRS field trial, treatment was effective if begun within the first 4 days of fever, and continued for a 7 day course. A compassionate use protocol, utilizing intravenous ribavirin as a treatment for Lassa fever, is sponsored by the CDC. Doses are slightly different, and continued for a 10 day course; treatment is most effective if begun within 7 days of onset. The only significant side effect of ribavirin is a modest anemia due to a reversible inhibition of erythropoiesis, and mild hemolysis. Although ribavirin is teratogenic in laboratory animals, the potential benefits must be weighed against the potential risks to pregnant women with grave illness due to one of these VHFs. Safety in infants and children has not been established. Ribavirin has poor *in vitro* and *in vivo* activity against the filoviruses (Ebola and Marburg) and the flaviviruses (dengue, yellow fever, Omsk HF and Kyanasur Forest Disease).

Argentine HF responds to therapy with 2 or more units of convalescent plasma containing adequate amounts of neutralizing antibody and given within 8 days of onset.

This therapy is investigational, and available only under protocol.

PROPHYLAXIS

The only licensed vaccine available for any of the hemorrhagic fever viruses is yellow fever vaccine, which is mandatory for travelers to endemic areas of Africa and South America. Argentine hemorrhagic fever vaccine is a live, attenuated, investigational vaccine developed at USAMRIID, which has proved efficacious both in an animal model and in a field trial in South America, and seems to protect against Bolivian hemorrhagic fever as well. Both inactivated and live-attenuated Rift Valley fever vaccines are currently under investigation. An investigational vaccinia-vectored Hantaan vaccine is offered to laboratory workers at USAMRIID. There are currently no vaccines for the other VHF agents available for human use in the United States.

Persons with percutaneous or mucocutaneous exposure to blood, body fluids, secretions, or excretions from a patient with suspected VHF should immediately wash the affected skin surfaces with soap and water. Mucous membranes should be irrigated with copious amounts of water or saline.

Close personal contacts or medical personnel exposed to blood or secretions from VHF patients (particularly Lassa fever, CCHF, and filoviral diseases) should be monitored for symptoms, fever and other signs during the established incubation period. A DoD compassionate use protocol exists for prophylactic administration of oral ribavirin to high risk contacts (direct exposure to body fluids) of Congo-Crimean HF patients. A similar post-exposure prophylaxis strategy has been suggested for high contacts of Lassa fever patients. Most patients will tolerate this dose well, but patients should be under surveillance for breakthrough disease (especially after drug cessation) or adverse drug effects (principally anemia).

ISOLATION AND CONTAINMENT

These viruses pose special challenges for hospital infection control. With the exception of dengue (virus present, but no secondary infection hazard) and hantaviruses (infectious virus not present in blood or excreta at the time of clinical presentation), VHF patients generally have significant quantities of virus in blood and often other secretions. Special caution must be exercised in handling sharps, needles, and other potential sources of parenteral exposure. Strict adherence to standard precautions will prevent nosocomial transmission of most VHFs.

Lassa, Congo-Crimean HF, Ebola, and Marburg viruses may be particularly prone to aerosol nosocomial spread. Secondary infections among contacts and medical personnel who were not parenterally exposed are well documented. Sometimes this occurred when the acute hemorrhagic disease (as seen in CCHF) mimicked a surgical emergency such as a bleeding gastric ulcer, with subsequent exposure and secondary spread among emergency and operating room personnel. Therefore, when one of these diseases is suspected, additional management measures are indicated. The patient should be hospitalized in a private room. An adjoining anteroom for putting on and removing protective barriers, storage of supplies, and decontamination of laboratory specimen containers, should be used if available. A room with non-recirculated air under negative pressure is advised for patients with significant cough, hemorrhage, or diarrhea. It may be wise to place the patient in such a room initially, to avoid having to transport the patient in the event of clinical deterioration. All persons entering the room should wear gloves and gowns (contact isolation). In addition, face shields or surgical masks and eye protection are indicated for those coming within three feet of the patient. Respiratory protection should be upgraded to airborne isolation, including the use of a fit-tested HEPA filtered respirator, a battery powered air purifying respirator, or a positive pressure supplied air respirator, if patients with the above conditions have prominent cough, vomiting, diarrhea, or hemorrhage. Caution should be exercised in evaluating and treating the patient with suspected VHF. Over-reaction on the part of health care providers is inappropriate and detrimental to both patient and staff, but it is prudent to provide as rigorous isolation measures as feasible.

Laboratory specimens should be double-bagged, and the exterior of the outer bag decontaminated prior to transport to the laboratory. Excreta and other contaminated materials should be autoclaved, or decontaminated by the liberal application of hypochlorite or phenolic disinfectants. Clinical laboratory personnel are also at risk for exposure, and should employ a biosafety cabinet (if available) and barrier precautions when handling specimens.

No carrier state has been observed for any VHF, but excretion of virus in urine (e.g., Lassa fever) or semen (e.g., Argentine hemorrhagic fever) may occur during convalescence. Should the patient die, there should be minimal handling of the body, with sealing of the corpse in leak-proof material for prompt burial or cremation.

BIOLOGICAL TOXINS

Toxins are harmful substances produced by living organisms (animals, plants, microbes). Features that distinguish them from chemical agents, such as VX, cyanide, or mustard, include being not man-made, non-volatile (no vapor hazard), usually not dermally active (mycotoxins are the exception), and generally much more toxic per weight than chemical agents. Their lack of volatility is very important and makes them unlikely to produce either secondary or person-to-person exposures, or a persistent environmental hazard.

A toxin's utility as an aerosol weapon is determined by its toxicity, stability, and ease of production. The bacterial toxins, such as botulinum toxins, are the most toxic substances by weight known (Appendix I). Less toxic compounds, such as the mycotoxins, are thousands of times less toxic than botulinum, and have limited aerosol potential. The relationship between aerosol toxicity and the quantity of toxin required for an effective open-air exposure is shown in Appendix J, which demonstrates that for some agents such as the mycotoxins and ricin, very large quantities (tons) would be needed for an effective open-air attack. Stability limits the open-air potential of some toxins. For example, botulinum and tetanus toxins are large molecular weight proteins, and are easily denatured by environmental factors (heat, dessication, UV light), thus posing little downwind threat. Finally, some toxins, such as saxitoxin, might be both stable and highly toxic, but are so difficult to extract that they can only feasibly be produced in minute quantities.

As with all biological weapons, potential to cause incapacitation as well as lethality must be considered. Depending on the goals of an adversary, incapacitating agents may be more effective than lethal agents due to the overwhelming demand on the medical and evacuation infrastructure, or the expected panic in the population. Several toxins such as SEB, cause significant illness at doses much lower than that required for lethality, and thus pose a significant incapacitating threat.

This manual will cover four toxins considered to be among the most likely to be used against U.S. military and civilian targets: botulinum toxins, ricin, staphylococcal enterotoxin B (SEB), and T-2 mycotoxins.

BOTULINUM

SUMMARY

Signs and Symptoms: Usually begins with cranial nerve palsies, including ptosis, blurred vision, diplopia, dry mouth and throat, dysphagia, and dysphonia. This is followed by symmetrical descending flaccid paralysis, with generalized weakness and progression to respiratory failure. Symptoms begin as early as 12-36 hours after inhalation, but may take several days after exposure to low doses of toxin.

Diagnosis: Diagnosis is primarily a clinical one. Biowarfare attack should be suspected if multiple casualties simultaneously present with progressive descending flaccid paralysis. Lab confirmation can be obtained by bioassay (mouse neutralization) of the patient's serum. Other helpful labs include: ELISA or ECL for antigen in environmental samples, PCR for bacterial DNA in environmental samples, or nerve conduction studies and electromyography.

Treatment: Early administration of trivalent licensed antitoxin or heptavalent antitoxin (IND product) may prevent or decrease progression to respiratory failure and hasten recovery. Intubation and ventilatory assistance for respiratory failure. Tracheostomy may be required.

Prophylaxis: Pentavalent toxoid vaccine (types A, B, C, D, and E) is available as an IND product for those at high risk of exposure.

Isolation and Decontamination: Standard Precautions for healthcare workers. Toxin is not dermally active and secondary aerosols are not a hazard from patients. Decon with soap and water. Botulinum toxin is inactivated by sunlight within 1-3 hours. Heat (80°C for 30 min., 100°C for several minutes) and chlorine (>99.7% inactivation by 3 mg/L FAC in 20 min.) also destroy the toxin.

OVERVIEW

The botulinum toxins are a group of seven related neurotoxins produced by the spore-forming bacillus *Clostridium botulinum* and two other *Clostridia* species. These toxins, types A through G, are the most potent neurotoxins known; paradoxically, they have been used therapeutically to treat spastic conditions (strabismus, blepharospasm, torticollis, tetanus) and cosmetically to treat wrinkles. The spores are ubiquitous; they germinate into vegetative bacteria that produce toxins during anaerobic incubation. Industrial-scale fermentation can produce large quantities of toxin for use as a BW agent. There are three epidemiologic forms of naturally occurring botulism—foodborne, infantile, and wound. Botulinum could be delivered by aerosol or used to contaminate food or water supplies. When inhaled, these toxins produce a clinical picture very similar to foodborne intoxication, although the time to onset of paralytic symptoms after inhalation may actually be longer than for foodborne cases, and may vary by type and dose of toxin. The clinical syndrome produced by these toxins is known as "botulism".

HISTORY AND SIGNIFICANCE

Botulinum toxins have caused numerous cases of botulism when ingested in improperly prepared or canned foods. Many deaths have occurred secondary to such incidents. It is feasible to deliver botulinum toxins as an aerosolized biological weapon, and several countries and terrorist groups have weaponized them. Botulinum toxins were weaponized by the U.S. in its old offensive BW program. Evidence obtained by the United Nations in 1995 revealed that Iraq had filled and deployed over 100 munitions with nearly 10,000 liters of botulinum toxin. The Aum Shinrikyo cult in Japan weaponized and attempted to disseminate botulinum toxin on multiple occasions in Tokyo prior to their 1995 Sarin attack in the Tokyo subway.

TOXIN CHARACTERISTICS

The botulinum toxins are the most toxic compounds, per weight of agent, known to man, requiring only 0.001 microgram per kilogram of body weight to kill 50 percent of the animals studied. Botulinum toxin type A is 15,000 times more toxic by weight than VX and 100,000 times more toxic than Sarin, two of the well-known organophosphate nerve agents.

Botulinum toxins are proteins with molecular weights of approximately 150,000 Daltons. Each of the seven distinct, but related neurotoxins, A through G, is produced by a different strain of *Clostridia*. All seven types act by the same mechanism. The toxins produce similar effects when inhaled or ingested, although the time course may vary depending on the route of exposure and the dose received. Although an aerosol attack is the most likely scenario for the use of botulinum toxins, the agent could be used to sabotage food supplies. Enemy special forces or terrorists might use this method in certain scenarios to produce foodborne botulism in specific targets.

These large proteins are easily denatured by environmental conditions. The toxins are detoxified in air within 12 hours. Sunlight inactivates the toxins within 1-3 hours. Heat destroys the toxins in 30 minutes at $80^{\circ}C$ and in several minutes at $100^{\circ}C$. In water, the toxins are >99.7% inactivated by 20 minutes' exposure to 3 mg/L free available chlorine (FAC), similar to the military disinfection procedure; and 84% inactivated by 20 minutes at 0.4% mg/L FAC, similar to municipal water treatment procedures.

MECHANISM OF TOXICITY

Botulinum toxin consists of two polypeptide subunits (A and B chains). The B subunit binds to receptors on the axons of motor neurons. The toxin is taken into the axon, where the A chain exerts its cytotoxic effect; it inactivates the axon, preventing release of acetylcholine and blocking neuromuscular transmission (pre-synaptic inhibition). Recovery follows only after the neuron develops a new axon, which can take months. The presynaptic inhibition affects both cholinergic autonomic (muscarinic) and motor (nicotinic) receptors. This interruption of neurotransmission causes cranial nerve and skeletal muscle paralysis seen in clinical botulism.

Unlike the situation with nerve agent intoxication, where there is too much acetylcholine due to inhibition of acetylcholinesterase, the problem in botulism is lack of the neurotransmitter in the synapse. Thus, pharmacologic measures such as atropine are not indicated in botulism and would likely exacerbate symptoms (see Appendix H).

CLINICAL FEATURES

The onset of symptoms of inhalation botulism usually occurs from 12 to 36 hours following exposure, but can vary according to the amount of toxin absorbed, and could be reduced following a BW attack. Recent primate studies indicate that the signs and symptoms may not appear for several days when a low dose of the toxin is inhaled versus a shorter time period following ingestion of toxin or inhalation of higher doses.

Cranial nerve palsies are prominent early, with eye symptoms such as blurred vision due to mydriasis, diplopia, ptosis, and photophobia, in addition to other cranial nerve signs such as dysarthria, dysphonia, and dysphagia. Flaccid skeletal muscle paralysis follows, in a symmetrical, descending, and progressive manner. Collapse of the upper airway may occur due to weakness of the oropharyngeal musculature. As the descending motor weakness involves the diaphragm and accessory muscles of respiration, respiratory failure may occur abruptly. Progression from onset of symptoms to respiratory failure has occurred in as little as 24 hours in cases of severe foodborne botulism.

The autonomic effects of botulism are manifested by typical anticholinergic signs and symptoms: dry mouth, ileus, constipation, and urinary retention. Nausea and vomiting may occur as nonspecific sequelae of an ileus. Dilated pupils (mydriasis) are seen in approximately 50 percent of cases.

Sensory symptoms usually do not occur. Botulinum toxins do not cross the blood/brain barrier and do not cause CNS disease. However, the psychological sequelae of botulism may be severe and require specific intervention.

Physical examination usually reveals an afebrile, alert, and oriented patient. Postural hypotension may be present. Mucous membranes may be dry and crusted and the patient may complain of dry mouth or sore throat. There may be difficulty with speaking and swallowing. Gag reflex may be absent. Pupils may be dilated and even fixed. Ptosis and extraocular muscle palsies may also be present. Variable degrees of skeletal muscle weakness may be observed depending on the degree of progression in an individual patient. Deep tendon reflexes may be present or absent. With severe respiratory muscle paralysis, the patient may become cyanotic or exhibit narcosis from CO_2 retention.

DIAGNOSIS

The occurrence of an epidemic of afebrile patients with progressive symmetrical descending flaccid paralysis strongly suggests botulinum intoxication. Foodborne outbreaks tend to occur in small clusters and have never occurred in soldiers on military rations such as MRE's (Meals, Ready to Eat). Higher numbers of cases in a theater of operations should raise at least the consideration of a biological warfare attack with aerosolized botulinum toxin.

Individual cases might be confused clinically with other neuromuscular disorders such as Guillain-Barre syndrome, myasthenia gravis, or tick paralysis. The edrophonium or Tensilon® test may be transiently positive in botulism, so it may not distinguish botulinum intoxication from myasthenia. The cerebrospinal fluid in botulism is normal and the paralysis is generally symmetrical, which distinguishes it from enteroviral myelitis. Mental status changes generally seen in viral encephalitis should not occur with botulinum intoxication.

It may become necessary to distinguish nerve agent and/or atropine poisoning from botulinum intoxication. Nerve agent poisoning produces copious respiratory secretions and miotic pupils, whereas a decrease in secretions is more likely in botulinum intoxication. Atropine overdose is distinguished from botulism by its central nervous system excitation (hallucinations and delirium) even though the mucous membranes are dry and mydriasis is present. The clinical differences between botulinum intoxication and nerve agent poisoning are depicted in Appendix H.

Laboratory testing is generally not critical to the diagnosis of botulism. Mouse neutralization (bioassay) remains the most sensitive test, and serum samples should be drawn and sent to a lab capable of this test. PCR might detect *C. botulinum* genes in an environmental sample. Detection of toxin in clinical or environmental samples is sometimes possible using an ELISA or ECL test. Clinical samples can include serum, gastric aspirates, stool, and respiratory secretions. Survivors do not usually develop an antibody response due to the very small amount of toxin necessary to produce clinical symptoms.

MEDICAL MANAGEMENT

Supportive care, including prompt respiratory support, can be lifesaving. Respiratory failure due to paralysis of respiratory muscles is the most serious effect and, generally, the cause of death. Reported cases of botulism prior to 1950 had a mortality rate of 60%. With tracheotomy or endotracheal intubation and ventilatory assistance, fatalities are less than five percent today. Prevention of nosocomial infections is a primary concern, along with hydration, nasogastric suctioning for ileus, bowel and bladder care, and prevention of decubitus ulcers and deep venous thromboses. Intensive and prolonged nursing care may be required for recovery, which may take up to three months for initial signs of improvement, and up to a year for complete resolution of symptoms.

Antitoxin: Early administration of botulinum antitoxin is critical, since the antitoxin can only neutralize the circulating toxin in patients with symptoms that continue to progress. When symptom progression ceases, no circulating toxin remains, and the antitoxin has no effect. Antitoxin may be particularly effective in food-borne cases, where presumably toxin continues to be absorbed through the gut wall. Animal experiments show that after aerosol exposure, botulinum antitoxin is very effective if given before the onset of clinical signs. If the antitoxin is delayed until after the onset of symptoms, it does not protect against respiratory failure.

Three different antitoxin preparations are available in the U.S. A licensed trivalent (types A, B, E) equine antitoxin is available from the Centers for Disease Control and Prevention for cases of foodborne botulism. This product has all the disadvantages of a horse serum product, including the risks of anaphylaxis and serum sickness. A monovalent human antiserum (type A) is available from the California Department of Health Services for infant botulism. A "despeciated" equine heptavalent antitoxin against all 7 serotypes has been prepared by cleaving the Fc fragments from horse IgG molecules, leaving $F(ab)_2$ fragments. This product was developed by USAMRIID, and is currently available under IND status. It has been effective in animal studies. However, 4% of horse antigens remain, so there is still a risk of hypersensitivity reactions.

Use of the equine antitoxin requires skin testing for horse serum sensitivity prior to administration. Skin testing is performed by injecting 0.1 ml of a 1:10 dilution (in sterile physiological saline) of antitoxin intradermally in the patient's forearm with a 26 or 27 gauge needle. Monitor the injection site and observe the patient for allergic reaction for 20 minutes. The skin test is positive if any of these allergic reactions occur: hyperemic areola at the site of the injection > 0.5 cm;

fever or chills; hypotension with decrease of blood pressure > 20 mm Hg for systolic and diastolic pressures; skin rash; respiratory difficulty; nausea or vomiting; generalized itching. Do NOT administer equine derived Botulinum F(ab')$_2$ Antitoxin if the skin test is positive. If no allergic symptoms are observed, the antitoxin is administered as a single dose intravenously in a normal saline solution, 10 ml over 20 minutes.

With a positive skin test, desensitization can be attempted by administering 0.01 - 0.1 ml of antitoxin subcutaneously, doubling the previous dose every 20 minutes until 1.0 - 2.0 ml can be sustained without any marked reaction. Preferably, desensitization should be performed by an experienced allergist. Medical personnel administering the antitoxin should be prepared to treat anaphylaxis with epinephrine, intubation equipment, and IV access.

PROPHYLAXIS

Vaccine: A pentavalent toxoid of *Clostridium botulinum* toxin types A, B, C, D, and E is available as an IND for pre-exposure prophylaxis. It will likely remain under IND status since efficacy testing in humans is not feasible. This product has been administered to several thousand volunteers and occupationally at-risk workers, and induces serum antitoxin levels that correspond to protective levels in experimental animals. The currently recommended primary series of 0, 2, and 12 weeks, followed by a 1 year booster induces protective antibody levels in greater than 90 percent of vaccinees after one year. Adequate antibody levels are transiently induced after three injections, but decline prior to the one year booster.

Contraindications to the vaccine include sensitivities to alum, formaldehyde, and thimerosal, or hypersensitivity to a previous dose. Reactogenicity is mild, with two to four percent of vaccinees reporting erythema, edema, or induration at the local site of injection which peaks at 24 to 48 hours. The frequency of such local reactions increases with subsequent inoculations; after the second and third doses, seven to ten percent will have local reactions, with higher incidence (up to twenty percent or so) after boosters. Severe local reactions are rare, consisting of more extensive edema or induration. Systemic reactions are reported in up to three percent, consisting of fever, malaise, headache, and myalgia. Incapacitating reactions (local or systemic) are uncommon. The vaccine should be stored at 2-8°C (not frozen).

The vaccine is recommended for selected individuals or groups judged at high risk for exposure to botulinum toxin aerosols. There is no indication at present for use of botulinum antitoxin as a prophylactic modality except under extremely specialized circumstances.

Post-exposure prophylaxis, using the heptavalent antitoxin has been demonstrated effective in animal studies; however, human data are not available, so it is not recommended for this indication. The antitoxin should be considered for this purpose only in extraordinary circumstances.

RICIN

SUMMARY

Signs and Symptoms: Acute onset of fever, chest tightness, cough, dyspnea, nausea, and arthralgias occurs 4 to 8 hours after inhalational exposure. Airway necrosis and pulmonary capillary leak resulting in pulmonary edema would likely occur within 18-24 hours, followed by severe respiratory distress and death from hypoxemia in 36-72 hours.

Diagnosis: Acute lung injury in large numbers of geographically clustered patients suggests exposure to aerosolized ricin. The rapid time course to severe symptoms and death would be unusual for infectious agents. Serum and respiratory secretions should be submitted for antigen detection (ELISA). Acute and convalescent sera provide retrospective diagnosis. Nonspecific laboratory and radiographic findings include leukocytosis and bilateral interstitial infiltrates.

Treatment: Management is supportive and should include treatment for pulmonary edema. Gastric lavage and cathartics are indicated for ingestion, but charcoal is of little value for large molecules such as ricin.

Prophylaxis: There is currently no vaccine or prophylactic antitoxin available for human use, although immunization appears promising in animal models. Use of the protective mask is currently the best protection against inhalation.

Isolation and Decontamination: Standard Precautions for healthcare workers. Ricin is non-volatile, and secondary aerosols are not expected to be a danger to health care providers. Decontaminate with soap and water. Hypochlorite solutions (0.1% sodium hypochlorite) can inactivate ricin.

OVERVIEW

Ricin is a potent protein cytotoxin derived from the beans of the castor plant (*Ricinus communis*). Castor beans are ubiquitous worldwide, and the toxin is fairly easy to extract; Therefore, ricin is potentially widely available. When inhaled as a small particle aerosol, this toxin may produce pathologic changes within 8 hours and severe respiratory symptoms followed by acute hypoxic respiratory failure in 36-72 hours. When ingested, ricin causes severe gastrointestinal symptoms followed by vascular collapse and death. This toxin may also cause disseminated intravascular coagulation, microcirculatory failure and multiple organ failure if given intravenously in laboratory animals.

HISTORY AND SIGNIFICANCE

Ricin's significance as a potential biological warfare toxin relates in part to its wide availability. Worldwide, one million tons of castor beans are processed annually in the production of castor oil; the waste mash from this process is 5% ricin by weight. The toxin is also quite stable and extremely toxic by several routes of exposure, including the respiratory route. Ricin was apparently used in the assassination of Bulgarian exile Georgi Markov in London in 1978. Markov was attacked with a specially engineered weapon disguised as an umbrella, which implanted a ricin-containing pellet into his body. This technique was used in at least six other assassination attempts in the late 1970's and early 1980's. In 1994 and 1995, four men from a tax-protest group known as the "Minnesota Patriots Council," were convicted of possessing ricin and conspiring to use it (by mixing it with the solvent DMSO) to murder law enforcement officials. In 1995, a Kansas City oncologist, Deborah Green, attempted to murder her husband by contaminating his food with ricin. In 1997, a Wisconsin resident, Thomas Leahy, was arrested and charged with possession with intent to use ricin as a weapon. Ricin has a high terrorist potential due to its ready availability, relative ease of extraction, and notoriety in the press.

TOXIN CHARACTERISTICS

Ricin is actually made up of two hemagglutinins and two toxins. The toxins, RCL III and RCL IV, are dimers with molecular weights of about 66,000 daltons. The toxins are made up of two polypeptide chains, an A chain and a B chain, which are joined by a disulfide bond. Ricin can be produced relatively easily and inexpensively in large quantities in a fairly low technology setting. Ricin can be prepared in liquid or crystalline form, or it can be lyophilized to make a dry powder. It could be disseminated as an aerosol, injected into a target, or used to contaminate food or water on a small scale. Ricin is stable under ambient conditions, but is detoxified by heat (80°C for 10 min., or 50°C for about an hour at pH 7.8) and chlorine (>99.4% inactivation by 100 mg/L FAC in 20 min.). Low chlorine concentrations, such as 10 mg/L FAC, as well as iodine at up to 16 mg/L, have no effect on ricin. Ricin's toxicity is marginal when comparing its LD50 to other toxins, such as botulinum and SEB (incapacitating dose). An enemy would need to produce it in large quantities to cover a significant area on the battlefield, thus potentially limiting large-scale use of ricin by an adversary.

MECHANISM OF TOXICITY

Ricin is very toxic to cells. It acts by inhibiting protein synthesis. The B chain binds to cell surface receptors and the toxin-receptor complex is taken into the cell; the A chain has endonuclease activity and extremely low concentrations will inhibit DNA replication and protein synthesis. In rodents, the histopathology of aerosol exposure is characterized by necrosis of upper and lower respiratory epithelium, causing tracheitis, bronchitis, bronchiolitis, and interstitial pneumonia with perivascular and alveolar edema. There is a latent period of 8 hours post-inhalation exposure before histologic lesions are observed in animal models. In rodents, ricin is more toxic by the aerosol route than by other routes of exposure.

CLINICAL FEATURES

The clinical picture in intoxicated victims would depend on the route of exposure. After aerosol exposure, signs and symptoms would depend on the dose inhaled. Accidental sublethal aerosol exposures which occurred in humans in the 1940's were characterized by acute onset of the following symptoms in 4 to 8 hours: fever, chest tightness, cough, dyspnea, nausea, and arthralgias. The onset of profuse sweating some hours later was commonly the sign of termination of most of the symptoms. Although lethal human aerosol exposures have not been described, the severe pathophysiologic changes seen in the animal respiratory tract, including necrosis and severe alveolar flooding, are probably sufficient to cause death from ARDS and respiratory failure. Time to death in experimental animals is dose dependent, occurring 36-72 hours post inhalation exposure. Humans would be expected to develop severe lung inflammation with progressive cough, dyspnea, cyanosis and pulmonary edema.

By other routes of exposure, ricin is not a direct lung irritant; however, intravascular injection can cause minimal pulmonary perivascular edema due to vascular endothelial injury. Ingestion causes necrosis of the gastrointestinal epithelium, local hemorrhage, and hepatic, splenic, and renal necrosis. Intramuscular injection causes severe local necrosis of muscle and regional lymph nodes with moderate visceral organ involvement.

DIAGNOSIS

An attack with aerosolized ricin would be primarily diagnosed by the clinical and epidemiological setting. Acute lung injury affecting a large number of geographically clustered cases should raise suspicion of an attack with a pulmonary irritant such as ricin, although other pulmonary pathogens could present with similar signs and symptoms. Other biological threats, such as SEB, Q fever, tularemia, plague, and some chemical warfare agents like phosgene, need to be included in the differential diagnosis. Ricin-induced pulmonary edema would be expected to occur much later (1-3 days post exposure) compared to that induced by SEB (about 12 hours post exposure) or phosgene (about 6 hours post exposure). Ricin intoxication would be expected to progress despite treatment with antibiotics, as opposed to an infectious process. There would be no mediastinitis as seen with inhalation anthrax. Ricin patients would not be expected to plateau clinically as occurs with SEB intoxication.

Specific ELISA and ECL testing on serum and respiratory secretions, or immunohistochemical stains of tissue may be used where available to confirm the diagnosis. Ricin is an extremely immunogenic toxin, and paired acute and convalescent sera should be obtained from survivors for measurement of antibody response. PCR can detect castor bean DNA in most ricin preparations. Additional supportive clinical or diagnostic features after aerosol exposure to ricin may include the following: bilateral infiltrates on chest radiographs, arterial hypoxemia, neutrophilic leukocytosis, and a bronchial aspirate rich in protein compared to plasma which is characteristic of high permeability pulmonary edema.

MEDICAL MANAGEMENT

Management of ricin-intoxicated patients depends on the route of exposure. Patients with pulmonary intoxication are managed by appropriate respiratory support (oxygen, intubation, ventilation, PEEP, and hemodynamic monitoring) and treatment for pulmonary edema, as indicated. Gastrointestinal intoxication is best managed by vigorous gastric lavage, followed by use of cathartics such as magnesium citrate. Superactivated charcoal is of little value for large molecules such as ricin. Volume replacement of GI fluid losses is important. In percutaneous exposures, treatment would be primarily supportive.

PROPHYLAXIS

The protective mask is effective in preventing aerosol exposure. Although a vaccine is not currently available, candidate vaccines are under development which are immunogenic and confer protection against lethal aerosol exposures in animals. Pre-exposure Prophylaxis with such a vaccine is the most promising defense against a biological warfare attack with ricin.

STAPHYLOCOCCAL ENTEROTOXIN B

SUMMARY

Signs and Symptoms: Latent period of 3-12 hours after aerosol exposure is followed by sudden onset of fever, chills, headache, myalgia, and nonproductive cough. Some patients may develop shortness of breath and retrosternal chest pain. Patients tend to plateau rapidly to a fairly stable clinical state. Fever may last 2 to 5 days, and cough may persist for up to 4 weeks. Patients may also present with nausea, vomiting, and diarrhea if they swallow the toxin. Presumably, higher exposure can lead to septic shock and death.

Diagnosis: Diagnosis is clinical. Patients present with a febrile respiratory syndrome without CXR abnormalities. Large numbers of patients presenting in a short period of time with typical symptoms and signs of SEB pulmonary exposure would suggest an intentional attack with this toxin.

Treatment: Treatment is limited to supportive care. Artificial ventilation might be needed for very severe cases, and attention to fluid management is important.

Prophylaxis: Use of protective mask. There is currently no human vaccine available to prevent SEB intoxication.

Isolation and Decontamination: Standard Precautions for healthcare workers. SEB is not dermally active and secondary aerosols are not a hazard from patients. Decon with soap and water. Destroy any food that may have been contaminated.

OVERVIEW

Staphylococcus aureus produces a number of exotoxins, one of which is Staphylococcal enterotoxin B, or SEB. Such toxins are referred to as exotoxins since they are excreted from the organism, and since they normally exert their effects on the intestines they are called enterotoxins. SEB is one of the pyrogenic toxins that commonly causes food poisoning in humans after the toxin is produced in improperly handled foodstuffs and subsequently ingested. SEB has a very broad spectrum of biological activity. This toxin causes a markedly different clinical syndrome when inhaled than it characteristically produces when ingested. Significant morbidity is produced in individuals who are exposed to SEB by either portal of entry to the body.

HISTORY AND SIGNIFICANCE

SEB is the second most common source of outbreaks of food poisoning. Often these outbreaks occur in a setting such as a church picnic or other community event, due to common source exposure in which contaminated food is consumed. Although an aerosolized SEB toxin weapon would not likely produce significant mortality, it could render 80 percent or more of exposed personnel clinically ill and unable to perform their mission for 1-2 weeks. The demand on the medical and logistical systems could be overwhelming. For these reasons, SEB was one of the 7 biological agents stockpiled by the U.S. during its old bioweapons program, which was terminated in 1969.

TOXIN CHARACTERISTICS

Staphylococcal enterotoxins are proteins of 23-29 kd molecular weight (SEB is 28,494). They are extracellular products of coagulase-positive staphylococci. Up to 50% of clinical isolates of *S. aureus* produce exotoxins. They are produced in culture media and also in foods when there is overgrowth of the staph organisms. Related toxins include toxic shock syndrome toxin-1 (TSST-1) and exfoliative toxins. SEB is one of at least seven antigenically distinct enterotoxins that have been identified. These toxins are moderately stable; SEB is inactivated after a few minutes at 100°C. SEB causes symptoms when inhaled at very low doses in humans: a dose of several logs lower (at least 100 times less) than the lethal dose by the inhaled route would be sufficient to incapacitate 50 percent of those exposed. This toxin could also be used to sabotage food or small volume water supplies.

MECHANISM OF TOXICITY

Staphylococcal enterotoxins belong to a class of potent immune stimulants known as bacterial superantigens. Superantigens bind to monocytes at major histocompatibility complex type II receptors rather than the usual antigen binding receptors. This leads to the direct stimulation of large populations of T-helper cells while bypassing the usual antigen processing and presentation. This induces a brisk cascade of pro-inflammatory cytokines (such as tumor necrosis factor, interferon, interleukin-1 and interleukin-2), with recruitment of other immune effector cells, and relatively deficient activation of counter-regulatory negative feedback loops. This results in an intense inflammatory response that injures host tissues. Released cytokines are thought to mediate many of the toxic effects of SEB.

CLINICAL FEATURES

Symptoms of SEB intoxication begin after a latent period of 3-12 hours after inhalation, or 4-10 hours after ingestion. Symptoms include nonspecific flu-like symptoms (fever, chills, headache, myalgias), and specific features dependent on the route of exposure. Oral exposure results in predominantly gastrointestinal symptoms: nausea, vomiting, and diarrhea. Inhalation exposures produce predominantly respiratory symptoms: nonproductive cough, retrosternal chest pain, and dyspnea. GI symptoms may accompany respiratory exposure due to inadvertent swallowing of the toxin after normal mucocilliary clearance.

Respiratory pathology is due to the activation of pro-inflammatory cytokine cascades in the lungs, leading to pulmonary capillary leak and pulmonary edema. Severe cases may result in acute pulmonary edema and respiratory failure.

The fever may last up to five days and range from 103 to 106 degrees F, with variable degrees of chills and prostration. The cough may persist up to four weeks, and patients may not be able to return to duty for two weeks.

Physical examination in patients with SEB intoxication is often unremarkable. Conjunctival injection may be present, and postural hypotension may develop due to fluid losses. Chest examination is unremarkable except in the unusual case where pulmonary edema develops. The chest X-ray is also generally normal, but in severe cases increased interstitial markings, atelectasis, and possibly overt pulmonary edema or an ARDS picture may develop.

DIAGNOSIS

Diagnosis of SEB intoxication is based on clinical and epidemiologic features. Because the symptoms of SEB intoxication may be similar to several respiratory pathogens such as influenza, adenovirus, and mycoplasma, the diagnosis may initially be unclear. All of these might present with fever, nonproductive cough, myalgia, and headache. SEB attack would cause cases to present in large numbers over a very short period of time, probably within a single 24-hour period. Naturally occurring pneumonias or influenza would involve patients presenting over a more prolonged interval of time. Naturally occurring staphylococcal food poisoning cases would not present with pulmonary symptoms. SEB intoxication tends to plateau rapidly to a fairly stable clinical state, whereas inhalational anthrax, tularemia pneumonia, or pneumonic plague would all continue to progress if left untreated. Tularemia and plague, as well as Q fever, would be associated with infiltrates on chest radiographs. Other diseases, including Hantavirus pulmonary syndrome, Chlamydia pneumonia, and CW agent inhalation (mustard, phosgene), should also be considered.

Laboratory confirmation of SEB intoxication includes antigen detection (ELISA, ECL) on environmental and clinical samples, and gene amplification (PCR – to detect *Staphylococcal* genes) on environmental samples. SEB may not be detectable in the serum by the time symptoms occur; regardless, a serum specimen should be drawn as early as possible after exposure. Data from rabbit studies clearly show that the presence of SEB in the serum is transient; however, it accumulates in the urine and can be detected for several hours post exposure. Therefore, urine samples should also be obtained and tested for SEB. Respiratory secretions and nasal swabs may demonstrate the toxin early (within 24 hours of exposure). Because most patients will develop a significant antibody response to the toxin, acute and convalescent sera should be drawn for retrospective diagnosis. Nonspecific findings include a neutrophilic leukocytosis, an elevated erythrocyte sedimentation rate, and chest x-ray abnormalities consistent with pulmonary edema.

MEDICAL MANAGEMENT

Currently, therapy is limited to supportive care. Close attention to oxygenation and hydration is important, and in severe cases with pulmonary edema, ventilation with positive end expiratory pressure, vasopressors and diuretics might be necessary. Acetaminophen for fever, and cough suppressants may make the patient more comfortable. The value of steroids is unknown. Most patients would be expected to do quite well after the initial acute phase of their illness, but generally would be unfit for duty for one to two weeks. Severe cases risk death from pulmonary edema and respiratory failure.

PROPHYLAXIS

Although there is currently no human vaccine for immunization against SEB intoxication, several vaccine candidates are in development. Preliminary animal studies have been encouraging. A vaccine candidate is nearing transition to advanced development for safety and immunogenicity testing in man. Experimentally, passive immunotherapy can reduce mortality in animals, but only when given within 4-8 hours after inhaling SEB. Because of the rapidity of SEB's binding with MHC receptors (<5 min. in vitro) active immunization is considered the most practical defense. Interestingly, most people have detectable antibody titers to SEB and SEC1, however, immunity acquired through natural exposure to SEB does not provide complete protection from an aerosol challenge (although it may reduce the emetic effect).

T-2 MYCOTOXINS

SUMMARY

Signs and symptoms: Exposure causes skin pain, pruritus, redness, vesicles, necrosis and sloughing of the epidermis. Effects on the airway include nose and throat pain, nasal discharge, itching and sneezing, cough, dyspnea, wheezing, chest pain and hemoptysis. Toxin also produces effects after ingestion or eye contact. Severe intoxication results in prostration, weakness, ataxia, collapse, shock, and death.

Diagnosis: Should be suspected if an aerosol attack occurs in the form of "yellow rain" with droplets of variously pigmented oily fluids contaminating clothes and the environment. Confirmation requires testing of blood, tissue and environmental samples.

Treatment: There is no specific antidote. Treatment is supportive. Soap and water washing, even 4-6 hours after exposure can significantly reduce dermal toxicity; washing within 1 hour may prevent toxicity entirely. Superactivated charcoal should be given orally if the toxin is swallowed.

Prophylaxis: The only defense is to prevent exposure by wearing a protective mask and clothing (or topical skin protectant) during an attack. No specific immunotherapy or chemotherapy is available for use in the field.

Isolation and Decontamination: Outer clothing should be removed and exposed skin decontaminated with soap and water. Eye exposure should be treated with copious saline irrigation. Secondary aerosols are not a hazard; however, contact with contaminated skin and clothing can produce secondary dermal exposures. Contact Precautions are warranted until decontamination is accomplished. Then, Standard Precautions are recommended for healthcare workers. Environmental decontamination requires the use of a hypochlorite solution under alkaline conditions such as 1% sodium hypochlorite and 0.1M NaOH with 1 hour contact time.

OVERVIEW

The trichothecene (T-2) mycotoxins are a group of over 40 compounds produced by fungi of the genus *Fusarium*, a common grain mold. They are small molecular weight compounds, and are extremely stable in the environment. They are the only class of toxin that is dermally active, causing blisters within a relatively short time after exposure (minutes to hours). Dermal, ocular, respiratory, and gastrointestinal exposures would be expected after an attack with mycotoxins.

HISTORY AND SIGNIFICANCE

The potential for use as a BW toxin was demonstrated to the Russian military shortly after World War II when flour contaminated with species of *Fusarium* was unknowingly baked into bread that was ingested by civilians. Some developed a protracted lethal illness called alimentary toxic aleukia (ATA) characterized by initial symptoms of abdominal pain, diarrhea, vomiting, prostration, and within days fever, chills, myalgias and bone marrow depression with granulocytopenia and secondary sepsis. Survival beyond this point allowed the development of painful pharyngeal/laryngeal ulceration and diffuse bleeding into the skin (petechiae and ecchymoses), melena, bloody diarrhea, hematuria, hematemesis, epistaxis and vaginal bleeding. Pancytopenia, and gastrointestinal ulceration and erosion were secondary to the ability of these toxins to profoundly arrest bone marrow and mucosal protein synthesis and cell cycle progression through DNA replication.

Mycotoxins allegedly were released from aircraft in the "yellow rain" incidents in Laos (1975-81), Kampuchea (1979-81), and Afghanistan (1979-81). It has been estimated that there were more than 6,300 deaths in Laos, 1,000 in Kampuchea, and 3,042 in Afghanistan. The alleged victims were usually unarmed civilians or guerrilla forces. These groups were not protected with masks or chemical protective clothing and had little or no capability of destroying the attacking enemy aircraft. These attacks were alleged to have occurred in remote jungle areas, which made confirmation of attacks and recovery of agent extremely difficult. Some investigators have claimed that the "yellow clouds" were, in fact, bee feces produced by swarms of migrating insects. Much controversy has centered upon the veracity of eyewitness and victim accounts, but there is evidence to make these allegations of BW agent use in these areas possible.

TOXIN CHARACTERISTICS

The trichothecene mycotoxins are low molecular weight (250-500 daltons) nonvolatile compounds produced by filamentous fungi (molds) of the genera *Fusarium*, *Myrotecium, Trichoderma, Stachybotrys* and others. The structures of approximately 150 trichothecene derivatives have been described in the literature. These substances are relatively insoluble in water but are highly soluble in ethanol, methanol and propylene glycol. The trichothecenes are extremely stable to heat and ultraviolet light inactivation. They retain their bioactivity even when autoclaved; heating to 1500° F for 30 minutes is required for inactivation. Hypochlorite solution alone is does not effectively inactivate the toxins. Rather, the addition of

0.1M NAOH to a 1% hypochlorite solution, with 1 hour contact time is required. Soap and water effectively remove this oily toxin from exposed skin or other surfaces.

MECHANISM OF TOXICITY

The mycotoxins appear to have multiple mechanisms of action, many of which are poorly understood. Their most notable effect stems from their ability to rapidly inhibit protein and nucleic acid synthesis. Thus, they are markedly cytotoxic to rapidly dividing cells such as in the bone marrow, GI tract (mucosal epithelium), skin, and germ cells. Since this imitates the hematopoietic and lymphoid effects of radiation sickness, the mycotoxins are referred to as "radiomimetic agents." The mycotoxins also alter cell membrane structure and function, inhibit mitochondrial respiration, and inactivate certain enzymes.

CLINICAL FEATURES

In a BW attack with trichothecenes, the toxin(s) can adhere to and penetrate the skin, be inhaled, and can be ingested. In the alleged yellow rain incidents, symptoms of exposure from all 3 routes coexisted. Contaminated clothing can serve as a reservoir for further toxin exposure. Early symptoms beginning within minutes of exposure include burning skin pain, redness, tenderness, blistering, and progression to skin necrosis with leathery blackening and sloughing of large areas of skin. Upper respiratory exposure may result in nasal itching, pain, sneezing, epistaxis, and rhinorrhea. Pulmonary/tracheobronchial toxicity produces dyspnea, wheezing, and cough. Mouth and throat exposure causes pain and blood tinged saliva and sputum. Anorexia, nausea, vomiting and watery or bloody diarrhea with crampy abdominal pain occurs with gastrointestinal toxicity. Eye pain, tearing, redness, foreign body sensation and blurred vision may follow ocular exposure. Skin symptoms occur in minutes to hours and eye symptoms in minutes. Systemic toxicity can occur via any route of exposure, and results in weakness, prostration, dizziness, ataxia, and loss of coordination. Tachycardia, hypothermia, and hypotension follow in fatal cases. Death may occur in minutes, hours or days. The most common symptoms are vomiting, diarrhea, skin involvement with burning pain, redness and pruritus, rash or blisters, bleeding, and dyspnea. A late effect of systemic absorption is pancytopenia, predisposing to bleeding and sepsis.

DIAGNOSIS

Clinical and epidemiological findings provide clues to the diagnosis. High attack rates, dead animals of multiple species, and physical evidence such as yellow, red, green, or other pigmented oily liquid are suggestive of mycotoxins. Rapid onset of symptoms in minutes to hours supports a diagnosis of a chemical or toxin attack. Mustard and other vesicant agents must be considered but they have an odor, are visible, and can be rapidly detected by a field chemical test (M8 paper, M256 kit). Symptoms from mustard toxicity are also delayed for several hours. Inhalation of staphylococcal enterotoxin B or ricin aerosols can cause fever, cough, dyspnea, and wheezing but does not involve the skin.

Specific diagnosis of T-2 mycotoxins in the form of a rapid diagnostic test is not presently available in the field. Serum and urine should be collected and sent to a reference lab for antigen detection. The mycotoxins and metabolites are eliminated in the urine and feces; 50-75% is eliminated within 24 hours, however, metabolites can be detected as late as 28 days after exposure. Pathologic specimens include blood, urine, lung, liver, and stomach contents. Environmental and clinical samples can be tested using a gas liquid chromatography-mass spectrometry technique. This system can detect as little as 0.1-1.0 ppb of T-2, which is sensitive enough to measure T-2 levels in the plasma of toxin victims.

MEDICAL MANAGEMENT

No specific antidote or therapeutic regimen is currently available. All therapy is supportive. If a soldier is unprotected during an attack the outer uniform should be removed within 4 hours and decontaminated by exposure to 5% hypochlorite for 6-10 hours. The skin should be thoroughly washed with soap and uncontaminated water if available. This can reduce dermal toxicity, even if delayed 4-6 hours after exposure. The M291 skin decontamination kit can also be used to remove skin-adherent T-2. Standard burn care is indicated for cutaneous involvement. Standard therapy for poison ingestion, including the use of superactivated charcoal to absorb swallowed T-2, should be administered to victims of an unprotected aerosol attack. Respiratory support may be necessary. The eyes should be irrigated with normal saline or water to remove toxin.

PROPHYLAXIS

Physical protection of the skin, mucous membranes, and airway (use of chemical protective mask and clothing) are the only proven effective methods of protection during an attack. Immunological (vaccines) and chemoprotective pretreatments are being studied in animal models, but are not available for field use by the warfighter. Topical skin protectant may limit dermal exposure. Soap and water washing, even 1 hour after dermal exposure to T-2, effectively prevents dermal toxicity.

DETECTION

Accurate intelligence is required to develop an effective defense against biological warfare. Once an agent has been dispersed, detection of the biological aerosol prior to its arrival over the target, in time for personnel to don protective equipment, is the best way to minimize or prevent casualties. However, interim systems for detecting biological agents are just now being fielded in limited numbers. Until reliable detectors are available in sufficient numbers, usually the first indication of a biological attack in unprotected soldiers will be the ill soldier.

Detector systems are evolving, and represent an area of intense interest with the highest priorities within the research and development community. Several systems are now being fielded. The Biological Integrated Detection System (BIDS) is vehicle- mounted and concentrates aerosol particles from environmental air, then subjects the particle sample to both genetic and antibody-based detection schemes for selected agents. The Long Range Biological Standoff Detection System (LRBSDS) will provide a first time biological standoff detection capability to provide early warning. It will employ infrared laser to detect aerosol clouds at a standoff distance up to 30 kilometers. An improved version is in development to extend the range to 100 km. This system will be available for fixed-site applications or inserted into various transport platforms such as fixed-wing or rotary aircraft. The Short-Range Biological Standoff Detection System (SRBSDS) is in the research and development phase. It will employ ultraviolet and laser-induced fluorescence to detect biological aerosol clouds at distances up to 5 kilometers. The information will be used to provide early warning, enhance contamination avoidance efforts, and cue other detection efforts.

The principal difficulty in detecting biological agent aerosols stems from differentiating the artificially generated BW cloud from the background of organic matter normally present in the atmosphere. Therefore, the aforementioned detection methods must be used in conjunction with intelligence, physical protection, and medical protection (vaccines and other chemoprophylactic measures) to provide layered primary defenses against a biological attack.

PERSONAL PROTECTION

The currently fielded chemical protective equipment, which includes the protective mask, battle dress overgarment (BDO), protective gloves, and overboots will provide protection against a biological agent attack.

The M40 protective mask is available in three sizes, and when worn correctly, will protect the face, eyes, and respiratory tract. The M40 utilizes a single screw-on filter element which involves two separate but complementary mechanisms: 1) impaction and adsorption of agent molecules onto ASC Whetlerite Carbon filtration media, and 2) static electrical attraction of particles initially failing to contact the filtration media. Proper maintenance and periodic replacement of the crucial filter elements are of the utmost priority. The filter MUST be replaced under these circumstances: the elements are immersed in water, crushed, cut, or otherwise damaged; excessive breathing resistance is encountered; the "ALL CLEAR" signal is given after exposure to a biological agent; 30 days have elapsed in the combat theater of operations (the filters must be replaced every 30 days); supply bulletins indicate lot number expiration; or when ordered by the unit commander. The filter element can only be changed in a non-contaminated environment. Two styles of optical inserts for the protective mask are available for soldiers requiring visual correction. The wire frame style is considered to be the safer of the two and is more easily fitted into the mask. A prong-type optical insert is also available. A drinking tube on the mask allows the wearer to drink while in a contaminated environment. Note that the wearer should disinfect the canteen and tube by wiping with a 5 percent hypochlorite solution before use.

The battle dress overgarment suits come in eight sizes and are currently available in both woodland and desert camouflage patterns. The suit may be worn for 24 continuous hours in a contaminated environment, but once contaminated, it must be replaced by using the MOPP-gear exchange procedure described in the Soldier's Manual of Common Tasks. The discarded BDO must be incinerated or buried. Chemical protective gloves and overboots come in various sizes and are both made from butyl rubber. They may be decontaminated and reissued. The gloves and overboots must be visually inspected and decontaminated as needed after every 12 hours of exposure in a contaminated environment. While the protective equipment will protect against biological agents, it is important to note that even standard uniform clothing of good quality affords a reasonable protection against dermal exposure of surfaces covered.

Those casualties unable to continue wearing protective equipment should be held and/or transported within casualty wraps designed to protect the patient against further chemical-biological agent exposure. Addition of a filter blower unit to provide overpressure enhances protection and provides cooling.

Collective protection by the use of either a hardened or unhardened shelter equipped with an air filtration unit providing overpressure can offer protection for personnel in the biologically contaminated environment. An airlock ensures that no contamination will be brought into the shelter. In the absence of a dedicated structure, enhanced protection can be afforded within most buildings by sealing cracks and entry ports, and providing air filtration with high efficiency particulate air (HEPA) filters within existing ventilation systems. The key problem is that these shelters can be very limited in military situations, very costly to produce and maintain, and difficult to deploy. Personnel must be decontaminated prior to entering the collective protection unit.

The most important route of exposure to biological agents is through inhalation. Biological warfare (BW) agents are dispersed as aerosols by one of two basic mechanisms: point or line source dissemination. Unlike some chemical threats, aerosols of agents disseminated by line source munitions (e.g., sprayed by low-flying aircraft or speedboats along the coast) do not leave hazardous environmental residua (although anthrax spores may persist and could pose a hazard near the dissemination line). On the other hand, aerosols generated by point-source munitions (i.e., stationary aerosol generator, bomblets, etc.) are more apt to produce ground contamination, but only in the immediate vicinity of dissemination. Point-source munitions leave an obvious signature that alerts the field commander that a biological warfare attack has occurred. Because point-source munitions always leave an agent residue, this evidence can be exploited for detection and identification purposes.

Aerosol delivery systems for biological warfare agents most commonly generate invisible clouds with particles or droplets of < 10 micrometers (μm). They can remain suspended for extensive periods. The major risk is pulmonary retention of inhaled particles. To a much lesser extent, particles may adhere to an individual or his clothing, thus the need for individual decontamination. The effective area covered varies with many factors, including wind speed, humidity, and sunlight. In the absence of an effective real-time alarm system or direct observation of an attack, the first clue would be mass casualties fitting a clinical pattern compatible with one of the biological agents. This may occur hours or days after the attack.

Toxins may cause direct pulmonary toxicity or be absorbed and cause systemic toxicity. Toxins are frequently as potent or more potent by inhalation than by any other route. A unique clinical picture may sometimes be seen which is not observed by other routes (e.g., pulmonary edema after staphylococcal enterotoxin B (SEB) exposure). Mucous membranes, including conjunctivae, are also vulnerable to many biological warfare agents. Physical protection is then quite important and the use of full-face masks equipped with small-particle filters, like the chemical protective masks, assumes a high degree of importance.

Other routes for delivery of biological agents are thought to be less important than inhalation, but are nonetheless potentially significant. Contamination of food and water supplies, either purposefully or incidentally after an aerosol biological warfare attack, represents a hazard for infection or intoxication by ingestion. Assurance that food and water supplies are free from contamination should be provided by appropriate preventive medicine authorities in the event of an attack.

Intact skin provides an excellent barrier for most biological agents. T-2 mycotoxins would be an exception because of their dermal activity. However, mucous membranes and abraded, or otherwise damaged, integument can allow for passage of some bacteria and toxins, and should be protected in the event of an attack.

DECONTAMINATION

Contamination is the introduction of an infectious agent on a body surface, food or water, or other inanimate objects. Decontamination involves either disinfection or sterilization to reduce microorganisms to an acceptable level on contaminated articles, thus rendering them suitable for use. Disinfection is the selective reduction of undesirable microbes to a level below that required for transmission. Sterilization is the killing of all organisms.

Decontamination methods have always played an important role in the control of infectious diseases. However, we are often unable use the most efficient means of rendering microbes harmless (e.g., toxic chemical sterilization), as these methods may injure people and damage materials which are to be decontaminated. BW agents can be decontaminated by mechanical, chemical and physical methods:

1) Mechanical decontamination involves measures to remove but not necessarily neutralize an agent. An example is the filtering of drinking water to remove certain water-borne pathogens (e.g. *Dracunculus medinensis*), or in a BW context, the use of an air filter to remove aerosolized anthrax spores, or water to wash agent from the skin.

2) Chemical decontamination renders BW agents harmless by the use of disinfectants that are usually in the form of a liquid, gas or aerosol. Some

161

disinfectants are harmful to humans, animals, the environment, and materials.

3) Physical means (heat, radiation) are other methods that can be employed for decontamination of objects.

Dermal exposure to a suspected BW aerosol should be immediately treated by soap and water decontamination. Careful washing with soap and water removes nearly all of the agent from the skin surface. Hypochlorite solution or other disinfectants are reserved for gross contamination (i.e. following the spill of solid or liquid agent from a munition directly onto the skin). In the absence of chemical or gross biological contamination, these will confer no additional benefit, may be caustic, and may predispose to colonization and resistant superinfection by reducing the normal skin flora. Grossly contaminated skin surfaces should be washed with a 0.5% sodium hypochlorite solution, if available, with a contact time of 10 to 15 minutes.

Ampules of calcium hypochlorite (HTH) are currently fielded in the Chemical Agent Decon Set for mixing hypochlorite solutions. The 0.5% solution can be made by adding one 6-ounce container of calcium hypochlorite to five gallons of water. The 5% solution can be made by adding eight 6-ounce ampules of calcium hypochlorite to five gallons of water. These solutions evaporate quickly at high temperatures so if they are made in advance they should be stored in closed containers. Also the chlorine solutions should be placed in distinctly marked containers because it is very

162

difficult to tell the difference between the 5% chlorine solution and the 0.5% solution.

To mix a 0.5% sodium hypochlorite solution, take one part Clorox and nine parts water (1:9) since standard stock Clorox is a 5.25% sodium hypochlorite solution. The solution is then applied with a cloth or swab. The solution should be made fresh daily with the pH in the alkaline range.

Chlorine solution must NOT be used in (1) open body cavity wounds, as it may lead to the formation of adhesions, or (2) brain and spinal cord injuries. However, this solution may be instilled into non-cavity wounds and then removed by suction to an appropriate disposal container. Within about 5 minutes, this contaminated solution will be neutralized and nonhazardous. Subsequent irrigation with saline or other surgical solutions should be performed. Prevent the chlorine solution from being sprayed into the eyes, as corneal opacities may result.

For decontamination of fabric clothing or equipment, a 5% hypochlorite solution should be used. For decontamination of equipment, a contact time of 30 minutes prior to normal cleaning is required. This is corrosive to most metals and injurious to most fabrics, so rinse thoroughly and oil metal surfaces after completion.

BW agents can be rendered harmless through such physical means as heat and radiation. To render agents completely harmless, sterilize with dry heat for two hours at 160 degrees centigrade. If autoclaving with steam at 121 degrees centigrade and 1 atmosphere of overpressure (15 pounds per square inch), the time may be reduced to 20 minutes, depending on volume. Solar ultraviolet (UV) radiation has a disinfectant effect, often in combination with drying. This is effective in certain environmental conditions but hard to standardize for practical usage for decontamination purposes.

The health hazards posed by environmental contamination by biological agents differ from those posed by persistent or volatile chemical agents. Aerosolized particles in the 1-5 µm size range will remain suspended due to brownian motion; suspended BW agents would be eventually inactivated by solar ultraviolet light, desiccation, and oxidation. Little, if any, environmental residues would occur. Possible exceptions include residua near the dissemination line, or in the immediate area surrounding a point-source munition. BW agents deposited on the soil would be subject to degradation by environmental stressors, and competing soil microflora. Simulant studies at Dugway Proving Ground suggest that secondary reaerosolization would be difficult, and would probably not pose a human health hazard. Environmental decontamination of terrain is costly and difficult and should be avoided, if possible. If grossly contaminated terrain, streets, or roads must be passed, the use of dust-binding spray to minimize reaerosolization may be considered. If it is necessary to decontaminate these surfaces, chlorine-calcium or lye may be used. Otherwise, rely on the natural processes which, especially outdoors, leads to the decontamination of agent by drying and solar UV radiation. Rooms in fixed spaces are best decontaminated with gases or liquids in aerosol form (e.g., formaldehyde). This is usually combined with surface disinfectants to ensure complete decontamination.

Appendix A: Glossary of Medical Terms

Adapted from Stedman's Electronic Medical Dictionary, Williams & Wilkins, Baltimore, MD, 1996 and Principles and Practice of Infectious Diseases, Mandell et al, Third Edition.

Acetylcholine (ACH, Ach) - The neurotransmitter substance at cholinergic synapses, which causes cardiac inhibition, vasodilation, gastrointestinal peristalsis, and other parasympathetic effects. It is liberated from preganglionic and postganglionic endings of parasympathetic fibers and from preganglionic fibers of the sympathetic as a result of nerve injuries, whereupon it acts as a transmitter on the effector organ; it is hydrolyzed into choline and acetic acid by acetylcholinesterase before a second impulse may be transmitted.

Active immunization -The act of artificially stimulating the body to develop antibodies against infectious disease by the administration of vaccines or toxoids.

Adenopathy - Swelling or morbid enlargement of the lymph nodes.

Aleukia - Absence or extremely decreased number of leukocytes in the circulating blood.

Analgesic - 1. A compound capable of producing analgesia, i.e., one that relieves pain by altering perception of nociceptive stimuli without producing anesthesia or loss of consciousness. 2. Characterized by reduced response to painful stimuli.

A-1

Anaphylaxis - The term is commonly used to denote the immediate, transient kind of immunologic (allergic) reaction characterized by contraction of smooth muscle and dilation of capillaries due to release of pharmacologically active substances (histamine, bradykinin, serotonin, and slow-reacting substance), classically initiated by the combination of antigen (allergen) with mast cell-fixed, cytophilic antibody (chiefly IgE).

Anticonvulsant - An agent which prevents or arrests seizures.

Antitoxin - An antibody formed in response to and capable of neutralizing a biological poison; an animal serum containing antitoxins.

Arthralgia - Severe pain in a joint, especially one not inflammatory in character.

AST - Abbreviation for aspartate aminotransferase, a liver enzyme.

Asthenia - Weakness or debility.

Ataxia - An inability to coordinate muscle activity during voluntary movement, so that smooth movements occur. Most often due to disorders of the cerebellum or the posterior columns of the spinal cord; may involve the limbs, head, or trunk.

Atelectasis - Absence of gas from a part or the whole of the lungs, due to failure of expansion or resorption of gas from the alveoli.

A-2

Atropine - An anticholinergic, with diverse effects (tachycardia, mydriasis, cycloplegia, constipation, urinary retention) attributable to reversible competitive blockade of acetylcholine at muscarinic type cholinergic receptors; used in the treatment of poisoning with organophosphate insecticides or nerve gases.

Bilirubin - A red bile pigment formed from hemoglobin during normal and abnormal destruction of erythrocytes. Excess bilirubin is associated with jaundice.

Blood agar - A mixture of blood and nutrient agar, used for the cultivation of many medically important microorganisms.

Bronchiolitis - Inflammation of the bronchioles, often associated with bronchopneumonia.

Bronchitis - Inflammation of the mucous membrane of the bronchial tubes.

Brucella - A genus of encapsulated, nonmotile bacteria (family Brucellaceae) containing short, rod-shaped to coccoid, Gram-negative cells. These organisms are parasitic, invading all animal tissues and causing infection of the genital organs, the mammary gland, and the respiratory and intestinal tracts, and are pathogenic for man and various species of domestic animals. They do not produce gas from carbohydrates.

Bubo - Inflammatory swelling of one or more lymph nodes, usually in the groin; the confluent mass of nodes usually suppurates and drains pus.

A-3

Bulla, gen. and pl. bullae - A large blister appearing as a circumscribed area of separation of the epidermis from the subepidermal structure (subepidermal *bulla*) or as a circumscribed area of separation of epidermal cells (intraepidermal *bulla*) caused by the presence of serum, or occasionally by an injected substance.

Carbuncle - Deep-seated pyogenic infection of the skin and subcutaneous tissues, usually arising in several contiguous hair follicles, with formation of connecting sinuses; often preceded or accompanied by fever, malaise, and prostration.

Cerebrospinal - Relating to the brain and the spinal cord.

Chemoprophylaxis - Prevention of disease by the use of chemicals or drugs.

Cholinergic - Relating to nerve cells or fibers that employ acetylcholine as their neurotransmitter.

CNS - Abbreviation for central nervous system.

Coagulopathy - A disease affecting the coagulability of the blood.

Coccobacillus - A short, thick bacterial rod of the shape of an oval or slightly elongated coccus.

Conjunctiva, pl. conjunctivae - The mucous membrane investing the anterior surface of the eyeball and the posterior surface of the lids.

A-4

CSF - Abbreviation for cerebrospinal fluid.

Cutaneous - Relating to the skin.

Cyanosis - A dark bluish or purplish coloration of the skin and mucous membrane due to deficient oxygenation of the blood, evident when reduced hemoglobin in the blood exceeds 5 g per 100 ml.

Diathesis -The constitutional or inborn state disposing to a disease, group of diseases, or metabolic or structural anomaly.

Diplopia -The condition in which a single object is perceived as two objects.

Distal - Situated away from the center of the body, or from the point of origin; specifically applied to the extremity or distant part of a limb or organ.

Dysarthria - A disturbance of speech and language due to emotional stress, to brain injury, or to paralysis, incoordination, or spasticity of the muscles used for speaking.

Dysphagia, dysphagy - Difficulty in swallowing.

Dysphonia - Altered voice production.

Dyspnea - Shortness of breath, a subjective difficulty or distress in breathing, usually associated with disease of the heart or lungs; occurs normally during intense physical exertion or at high altitude.

A-5

Ecchymosis - A purplish patch caused by extravasation of blood into the skin, differing from petechiae only in size (larger than 3 mm diameter).

Eczema - Generic term for inflammatory conditions of the skin, particularly with vesiculation in the acute stage, typically erythematous, edematous, papular, and crusting; followed often by lichenification and scaling and occasionally by duskiness of the erythema and, infrequently, hyperpigmentation; often accompanied by sensations of itching and burning.

Edema - An accumulation of an excessive amount of watery fluid in cells, tissues, or serous cavities.

Enanthem, enanthema - A mucous membrane eruption, especially one occurring in connection with one of the exanthemas.

Encephalitis, pl. encephalitides - Inflammation of the brain.

Endotoxemia - Presence in the blood of endotoxins.

Endotracheal intubation - Passage of a tube through the nose or mouth into the trachea for maintenance of the airway during anesthesia or for maintenance of an imperiled airway.

Enterotoxin - A cytotoxin specific for the cells of the intestinal mucosa.

Epistaxis - Profuse bleeding from the nose.

A-6

Epizootic - 1. Denoting a temporal pattern of disease occurrence in an animal population in which the disease occurs with a frequency clearly in excess of the expected frequency in that population during a given time interval. 2. An outbreak (epidemic) of disease in an animal population; often with the implication that it may also affect human populations.

Erythema - Redness of the skin due to capillary dilatation.

Erythema multiforme - An acute eruption of macules, papules, or subdermal vesicles presenting a multiform appearance, the characteristic lesion being the target or iris lesion over the dorsal aspect of the hands and forearms; its origin may be allergic, seasonal, or from drug sensitivity, and the eruption, although usually self-limited (e.g., multiforme minor), may be recurrent or may run a severe course, sometimes with fatal termination (e.g., multiforme major or Stevens-Johnson syndrome).

Erythrocyte - A mature red blood cell.

Erythropoiesis - The formation of red blood cells.

Exanthema - A skin eruption occurring as a symptom of an acute viral or coccal disease, as in scarlet fever or measles.

Extracellular -Outside tho cells.

Extraocular - Adjacent to but outside the eyeball.

Fasciculation - Involuntary contractions, or twitchings, of groups (fasciculi) of muscle fibers, a coarser form of muscular contraction than fibrillation.

Febrile - Denoting or relating to fever.

Fomite - Objects, such as clothing, towels, and utensils that possibly harbor a disease agent and are capable of transmitting it.

Formalin - A 37% aqueous solution of formaldehyde.

Fulminant hepatitis - Severe, rapidly progressive loss of hepatic function due to viral infection or other cause of inflammatory destruction of liver tissue.

Generalized vaccinia - Secondary lesions of the skin following vaccination which may occur in subjects with previously healthy skin but are more common in the case of traumatized skin, especially in the case of eczema (eczema vaccinatum). In the latter instance, generalized vaccinia may result from mere contact with a vaccinated person. Secondary vaccinial lesions may also occur following transfer of virus from the vaccination to another site by means of the fingers (autoinnoculation).

Glanders - A chronic debilitating disease of horses and other equids, as well as some members of the cat family, caused by *Pseudomonas mallei*; it is transmissible to humans. It attacks the mucous membranes of the nostrils of the horse, producing an increased and vitiated secretion and discharge of mucus, and enlargement and induration of the glands of the lower jaw.

Granulocytopenia -Less than the normal number of granular leukocytes in the blood.

Guarnieri bodies - Intracytoplasmic acidophilic inclusion body's observed in epithelial cells in variola (smallpox) and vaccinia infections, and which include aggregations of Paschen body's or virus particles.

Hemagglutination - The agglutination of red blood cells; may be immune as a result of specific antibody either for red blood cell antigens per se or other antigens which coat the red blood cells, or may be nonimmune as in hemagglutination caused by viruses or other microbes.

Hemagglutinin - A substance, antibody or other, that causes hemagglutination.

Hematemesis - Vomiting of blood.

Hemopoietic - Pertaining to or related to the formation of blood cells.

Hematuria - Any condition in which the urine contains blood or red blood cells.

Hemodynamic - Relating to the physical aspects of the blood circulation.

Hemolysis -Alteration, dissolution, or destruction of red blood cells in such a manner that hemoglobin is liberated into the medium in which the cells are suspended, e.g., by specific complement-fixing antibodies, toxins, various chemical agents, tonicity, alteration of temperature.

Hemolytic Uremic Syndrome - Hemolytic anemia and thrombocytopenia occurring with acute renal failure.

Hemoptysis - The spitting of blood derived from the lungs or bronchial tubes as a result of pulmonary or bronchial hemorrhage.

Hepatic - Relating to the liver.

Heterologous - 1. Pertaining to cytologic or histologic elements occurring where they are not normally found. 2. Derived from an animal of a different species, as the serum of a horse is heterologous for a rabbit.

Hyperemia - The presence of an increased amount of blood in a part or organ.

Hyperesthesia - Abnormal acuteness of sensitivity to touch, pain, or other sensory stimuli.

Hypotension - Subnormal arterial blood pressure.

Hypovolemia - A decreased amount of blood in the body.

Hypoxemia - Subnormal oxygenation of arterial blood, short of anoxia.

Idiopathic - Denoting a disease of unknown cause.

Immunoassay - Detection and assay of substances by serological (immunological) methods; in most applications the substance in question serves as antigen, both in antibody production and in measurement of antibody by the test substance.

A-10

In vitro - In an artificial environment, referring to a process or reaction occurring therein, as in a test tube or culture media.

In vivo - In the living body, referring to a process or reaction occurring therein.

Induration - 1. The process of becoming extremely firm or hard, or having such physical features. 2. A focus or region of indurated tissue.

Inguinal - Relating to the groin.

Inoculation - Introduction into the body of the causative organism of a disease.

Leukopenia - The antithesis of leukocytosis; any situation in which the total number of leukocytes in the circulating blood is less than normal, the lower limit of which is generally regarded as 4000-5000 per cu mm.

Lumbosacral - Relating to the lumbar vertebrae and the sacrum.

Lumen, pl. lumina - The space in the interior of a tubular structure, such as an artery or the intestine.

Lymphadenopathy - Any disease process affecting a lymph node or lymph nodes.

Lymphopenia - A reduction, relative or absolute, in the number of lymphocytes in the circulating blood.

Macula, pl. maculae - 1. A small spot, perceptibly different in color from the surrounding tissue. 2. A small, discolored patch or spot on the skin, neither elevated above nor depressed below the skin's surface.

Mediastinitis - Inflammation of the cellular tissue of the mediastinum.

Mediastinum - The median partition of the thoracic cavity, covered by the mediastinal pleura and containing all the thoracic viscera and structures except the lungs.

Megakaryocyte - A large cell with a polyploid nucleus that is usually multilobed; megakaryocytes are normally present in bone marrow, not in the circulating blood, and give rise to blood platelets.

Melena - Passage of dark-colored, tarry stools, due to the presence of blood altered by the intestinal juices.

Meningism - A condition in which the symptoms simulate a meningitis, but in which no actual inflammation of these membranes is present.

Meningococcemia - Presence of meningococci (*N. meningitidis*) in the circulating blood.

Meninges - Any membrane; specifically, one of the membranous coverings of the brain and spinal cord.

Microcyst - A tiny cyst, frequently of such dimensions that a magnifying lens or microscope is required for observation.

A-12

Microscopy - Investigation of minute objects by means of a microscope.

Moribund - Dying; at the point of death.

Mucocutaneous - Relating to mucous membrane and skin; denoting the line of junction of the two at the nasal, oral, vaginal, and anal orifices.

Myalgia - Muscular pain.

Mydriasis - Dilation of the pupil.

Narcosis - General and nonspecific reversible depression of neuronal excitability, produced by a number of physical and chemical agents, usually resulting in stupor rather than in anesthesia.

Necrosis - Pathologic death of one or more cells, or of a portion of tissue or organ, resulting from irreversible damage.

Nephropathia epidemica - A generally benign form of epidemic hemorrhagic fever reported in Scandinavia.

Neutrophilia - An increase of neutrophilic leukocytes in blood or tissues; also frequently used synonymously with leukocytosis, inasmuch as the latter is generally the result of an increased number of neutrophilic granulocytes in the circulating blood (or in the tissues, or both).

Nosocomial - Denoting a new disorder (not the patient's original condition) associated with being treated in a hospital, such as a hospital-acquired infection.

Oliguria - Scanty urine production.

Oropharynx - The portion of the pharynx that lies posterior to the mouth; it is continuous above with the nasopharynx via the pharyngeal isthmus and below with the laryngopharynx.

Osteomyelitis - Inflammation of the bone marrow and adjacent bone.

Pancytopenia - Pronounced reduction in the number of erythrocytes, all types of white blood cells, and the blood platelets in the circulating blood.

Pandemic - Denoting a disease affecting or attacking the population of an extensive region, country, continent; extensively epidemic.

Papule - A small, circumscribed, solid elevation on the skin.

Parasitemia -The presence of parasites in the circulating blood; used especially with reference to malarial and other protozoan forms, and microfilariae.

Passive immunity - Providing temporary protection from disease through the administration of exogenously produced antibody (i.e., transplacental transmission of antibodies to the fetus or the injection of immune globulin for specific preventive purposes).

PCR - see below for polymerase chain reaction.

A-14

Percutaneous - Denoting the passage of substances through unbroken skin, for example, by needle puncture, including introduction of wires and catheters.

Perivascular - Surrounding a blood or lymph vessel.

Petechia, pl. petechiae - Minute hemorrhagic spots, of pinpoint to pinhead size, in the skin, which are not blanched by pressure.

Pharyngeal - Relating to the pharynx.

Pharyngitis - Inflammation of the mucous membrane and underlying parts of the pharynx.

Phosgene - Carbonyl chloride; a colorless liquid below 8.2°C, but an extremely poisonous gas at ordinary temperatures; it is an insidious gas, since it is not immediately irritating, even when fatal concentrations are inhaled.

Photophobia - Morbid dread and avoidance of light. Photosensitivity, or pain in the eyes with exposure to light, can be a cause.

Pleurisy - Inflammation of the pleura.

Polymerase chain reaction - An in vitro method for enzymatically synthesizing and amplifying defined sequences of DNA in molecular biology. Can be used for improving DNA-based diagnostic procedures for identifying unknown BW agents.

Polymorphonuclear - Having nuclei of varied forms; denoting a variety of leukocyte.

Polyuria - Excessive excretion of urine.

Presynaptic - Pertaining to the area on the proximal side of a synaptic cleft.

Prophylaxis, pl. prophylaxes - Prevention of disease or of a process that can lead to disease.

Prostration - A marked loss of strength, as in exhaustion.

Proteinuria - Presence of urinary protein in concentrations greater than 0.3 g in a 24-hour urine collection or in concentrations greater than 1 g/l in a random urine collection on two or more occasions at least 6 hours apart; specimens must be clean, voided midstream, or obtained by catheterization.

Pruritus - Syn: itching.

Ptosis, pl. ptoses - In reference to the eyes, drooping of the eyelids.

Pulmonary edema -Edema of the lungs.

Pyrogenic - Causing fever.

Retinitis - Inflammation of the retina.

Retrosternal - Posterior to the sternum.

Rhinorrhea - A discharge from the nasal mucous membrane.

Sarin - A nerve poison which is a very potent irreversible cholinesterase inhibitor and a more toxic nerve gas than tabun or soman.

Scarification -The making of a number of superficial incisions in the skin. It is the technique used to administer tularemia and smallpox vaccines.

Septic shock - 1. shock associated with sepsis, usually associated with abdominal and pelvic infection complicating trauma or operations; 2. shock associated with septicemia caused by Gram-negative bacteria.

Sequela, pl. sequelae - A condition following as a consequence of a disease.

Shigellosis - Bacillary dysentery caused by bacteria of the genus *Shigella*, often occurring in epidemic patterns.

Soman - An extremely potent cholinesterase inhibitor, similar to sarin and tabun.

Sterile abscess - An abscess whose contents are not caused by pyogenic bacteria.

Stridor - A high-pitched, noisy respiration, like the blowing of the wind; a sign of respiratory obstruction, especially in the trachea or larynx.

Superantigen - An antigen that interacts with the T cell receptor in a domain outside of the antigen recognition site. This type of interaction induces the activation of larger numbers of T cells compared to antigens that are presented in the antigen recognition site.

Superinfection - A new infection in addition to one already present.

Tachycardia - Rapid beating of the heart, conventionally applied to rates over 100 per minute.

Teratogenicity -The property or capability of producing fetal malformation.

Thrombocytopenia - A condition in which there is an abnormally small number of platelets in the circulating blood.

Toxoid - A modified bacterial toxin that has been rendered nontoxic (commonly with formaldehyde) but retains the ability to stimulate the formation of antitoxins (antibodies) and thus producing an active immunity. Examples include Botulinum, tetanus, and diphtheria toxoids.

Tracheitis - Inflammation of the lining membrane of the trachea.

Urticaria - An eruption of itching wheals, usually of systemic origin; it may be due to a state of hypersensitivity to foods or drugs, foci of infection, physical agents (heat, cold, light, friction), or psychic stimuli.

Vaccine - A suspension of attenuated live or killed microorganisms (bacteria, viruses, or rickettsiae), or fractions thereof, administered to induce immunity and thereby prevent infectious disease.

Vaccinia - An infection, primarily local and limited to the site of inoculation, induced in man by inoculation with the vaccinia (coxpox) virus in order to confer resistance to smallpox (variola). On about the third day after vaccination, papules form at the site of inoculation which become transformed into umbilicated vesicles and later pustules; they then dry up, and the scab falls off on about the 21st day, leaving a pitted scar; in some cases there are more or less marked constitutional disturbances.

Varicella - An acute contagious disease, usually occurring in children, caused by the varicella-zoster virus, a member of the family *Herpesviridae*, and marked by a sparse eruption of papules, which become vesicles and then pustules, like that of smallpox although less severe and varying in stages, usually with mild constitutional symptoms; incubation period is about 14 to 17 days. Syn: chickenpox

Variola - Syn: smallpox.

Variolation - The historical practice of inducing immunity against smallpox by "scratching" the skin with the purulency from smallpox skin pustules. The first inoculation for smallpox is said to have been done in China about 1022 B.C.

Viremia - The presence of virus in the bloodstream.

Virion - The complete virus particle that is structurally intact and infectious.

Zoonosis - An infection or infestation shared in nature by humans and other animals that are the normal or usual host; a disease of humans acquired from an animal source.

Appendix B: Patient Isolation Precautions

Standard Precautions

- Wash hands after patient contact.
- Wear gloves when touching blood, body fluids, secretions, excretions and contaminated items.
- Wear a mask and eye protection, or a face shield during procedures likely to generate splashes or sprays of blood, body fluids, secretions or excretions
- Handle used patient-care equipment and linen in a manner that prevents the transfer of microorganisms to people or equipment.

Use care when handling sharps and use a mouthpiece or other ventilation device as an alternative to mouth-to-mouth resuscitation when practical.

Standard precautions are employed in the care of ALL patients

Airborne Precautions

Standard Precautions plus:
- Place the patient in a private room that has monitored negative air pressure, a minimum of six air changes/hour, and appropriate filtration of air before it is discharged from the room.
- Wear respiratory protection when entering the room.
- Limit movement and transport of the patient. Place a mask on the patient if they need to be moved.

Conventional Diseases requiring Airborne Precautions: Measles, Varicella, Pulmonary Tuberculosis.
Biothreat Diseases requiring Airborne Precautions: Smallpox.

B-1

Droplet Precautions

Standard Precaution plus:
- Place the patient in a private room or cohort them with someone with the same infection. If not feasible, maintain at least 3 feet between patients.
- Wear a mask when working within 3 feet of the patient.
- Limit movement and transport of the patient. Place a mask on the patient if they need to be moved.

Conventional Diseases requiring Droplet Precautions: Invasive *Haemophilus influenzae* and meningococcal disease, drug-resistant pneumococcal disease, diphtheria, pertussis, mycoplasma, GABHS, influenza, mumps, rubella, parvovirus.
Biothreat Diseases requiring Droplet precautions: Pneumonic Plague.

Contact Precautions

Standard Precautions plus:
- Place the patient in a private room or cohort them with someone with the same infection if possible.
- Wear gloves when entering the room. Change gloves after contact with infective material.
- Wear a gown when entering the room if contact with patient is anticipated or if the patient has diarrhea, a colostomy or wound drainage not covered by a dressing.

B-2

- Limit the movement or transport of the patient from the room.
- Ensure that patient-care items, bedside equipment, and frequently touched surfaces receive daily cleaning.
- Dedicate use of noncritical patient-care equipment (such as stethoscopes) to a single patient, or cohort of patients with the same pathogen. If not feasible, adequate disinfection between patients is necessary.

Conventional Diseases requiring Contact Precautions: MRSA, VRE, *Clostridium difficile*, RSV, parainfluenza, enteroviruses, enteric infections in the incontinent host, skin infections (SSSS, HSV, impetigo, lice, scabies), hemorrhagic conjunctivitis.

Biothreat Diseases requiring Contact Precautions: Viral Hemorrhagic Fevers.

For more information, see: Garner JS. Guideline for Infection Control Practices in Hospitals. Infect Control Hosp Epidemiol 1996;17:53-80.

Appendix C: BW Agent Characteristics

Disease	Transmit Man to Man	Infective Dose (Aerosol)	Incubation Period	Duration of Illness	Lethality (approx. case fatality rates)	Persistence of Organism	Vaccine Efficacy (aerosol exposure)
Inhalation anthrax	No	8,000-50,000 spores	1-6 days	3-5 days (usually fatal if untreated)	High	Very stable - spores remain viable for > 40 years in soil	2 dose efficacy against up to 1,000 LD_{50} in monkeys
Brucellosis	No	10 -100 organisms	5-60 days (usually 1-2 months)	Weeks to months	<5% untreated	Very stable	No vaccine
Cholera	Rare	10-500 organisms	4 hours - 5 days (usually 2-3 days)	≥ 1 week	Low with treatment, high without	Unstable in aerosols & fresh water; stable in salt water	No data on aerosol
Glanders	Low	Assumed low	10-14 days via aerosol	Death in 7-10 days in septicemic form	> 50%	Very stable	No vaccine
Pneumonic Plague	High	100-500 organisms	2-3 days	1-6 days (usually fatal)	High unless treated within 12-24 hours	For up to 1 year in soil; 270 days in live tissue	3 doses not protective against 118 LD_{50} in monkeys
Tularemia	No	10-50 organisms	2-10 days (average 3-5)	≥ 2 weeks	Moderate if untreated	For months in moist soil or other media	80% protection against 1-10 LD_{50}
Q Fever	Rare	1-10 organisms	10-40 days	2-14 days	Very low	For months on wood and sand	94% protection against 3,500 LD_{50} in guinea pigs

Appendix C: BW Agent Characteristics (Continued)

Disease	Transmit Man to Man	Infective Dose (Aerosol)	Incubation Period	Duration of Illness	Lethality (approx. case fatality rates)	Persistence of Organism	Vaccine Efficacy (aerosol exposure)
Smallpox	High	Assumed low (10-100 organisms)	7-17 days (average 12)	4 weeks	High to moderate	Very stable	Vaccine protects against large doses in primates
Venezuelan Equine Encephalitis	Low	10-100 organisms	2-6 days	Days to weeks	Low	Relatively unstable	TC 83 protects against 30-500 LD_{50} in hamsters
Viral Hemorrhagic Fevers	Moderate	1-10 organisms	4-21 days	Death between 7-16 days	High for Zaire strain, moderate with Sudan	Relatively unstable - depends on agent	No vaccine
Botulism	No	0.001 $\mu g/kg$ is LD_{50} for type A	1-5 days	Death in 24-72 hours; lasts months if not lethal	High without respiratory support	For weeks in nonmoving water and food	3 dose efficacy 100% against 25-250 LD_{50} in primates
Staph Enterotoxin B	No	0.03 μg/person incapacitation	3-12 hours after inhalation	Hours	< 1%	Resistant to freezing	No vaccine
Ricin	No	3-5 $\mu g/kg$ is LD_{50} in mice	18-24 hours	Days - death within 10-12 days for ingestion	High	Stable	No vaccine
T-2 Mycotoxins	No	Moderate	2-4 hours	Days to months	Moderate	For years at room temperature	No vaccine

Appendix D: BW Agents - Vaccine, Therapeutics, and Prophylaxis

DISEASE	VACCINE	CHEMOTHERAPY (Rx)	CHEMOPROPHYLAXIS (Px)	COMMENTS
Anthrax	Bioport vaccine (licensed) 0.5 mL SC @ 0, 2, 4 wk, 6, 12, 18 mo then annual boosters	Ciprofloxacin 400 mg IV q 12 h or Doxycycline 200 mg IV, then 100 mg IV q 12 h	Ciprofloxacin 500 mg PO bid x 4 wk If unvaccinated, begin initial doses of vaccine	Potential alternates for Rx: gentamicin, erythromycin, and chloramphenicol
		Penicillin 4 million units IV q 4 h	Doxycycline 100 mg PO bid x 4 wk plus vaccination	PCN for sensitive organisms only
Cholera	Wyeth-Ayerst Vaccine 2 doses 0.5 mL IM or SC @ 0, 7-30 days, then boosters Q 6 months	Oral rehydration therapy during period of high fluid loss	NA	Vaccine not recommended for routine protection in endemic areas (50% efficacy, short term)
		Tetracycline 500 mg q 6 h x 3 d		Alternates for Rx: erythromycin, trimethoprim and sulfamethoxazole, and furazolidone
		Doxycycline 300 mg once, or 100 mg q 12 h x 3 d		
		Ciprofloxacin 500 mg q 12 h x 3 d		Quinolones for tetra/doxy resistant strains
		Norfloxacin 400 mg q 12 h x 3 d		
Q Fever	IND 610 - inactivated whole cell vaccine given as single 0.5 ml s.c. injection	Tetracycline 500 mg PO q 6 h x 5-7 d continued at least 2 d after afebrile	Tetracycline 500 mg PO qid x 5 d (start 8-12 d post-exposure)	Currently testing vaccine to determine the necessity of skin testing prior to use.
		Doxycycline 100 mg PO q 12 h x 5-7 d continued at least 2 d after afebrile	Doxycycline 100 mg PO bid x 5 d (start 8-12 d post-exposure)	
Glanders	No vaccine available	Antibiotic regimens vary depending on localization and severity of disease - refer to text	Post-exposure prophylaxis may be tried with TMP-SMX	No large therapeutic human trials have been conducted owing to the rarity of naturally occurring disease.

Appendix D: BW Agents - Vaccine, Therapeutics, and Prophylaxis (Continued)

DISEASE	VACCINE	CHEMOTHERAPY (Rx)	CHEMOPROPHYLAXIS (Px)	COMMENTS
Plague	Greer inactivated vaccine (FDA licensed) is no longer available.	Streptomycin 30 mg/kg/d IM in 2 divided doses x 10 – 14 d or Gentamicin 5mg/kg or IV once daily x 10 - 14 d or Ciprofloxacin 400mg IV q 12 h until clinically improved then 750 mg PO bid for total of 10 – 14 d	Doxycycline 100 mg PO bid x 7 d or duration of exposure Ciprofloxacin 500 mg PO bid x 7 d	Chloramphenicol for plague meningitis is required 25 mg/kg IV, then 15 mg/kg qid x 14 d
		Doxycycline 200 mg IV then 100 mg IV bid, until clinically improved then 100mg PO bid for total of 10-14 d	Tetracycline 500 mg PO qid x 7 d	Alternate Rx: trimethoprim-sulfamethoxazole
Brucellosis	No human vaccine available	Doxycycline 200 mg/d PO plus rifampin 600 mg/d PO x 6 wk	Doxycycline 200 mg/d PO plus rifampin 600 mg/d PO x 6 wk	Trimethoprim-sulfamethoxazole may be substituted for rifampin; however, relapse may reach 30%
		Ofloxacin 400/rifampin 600 mg/d PO x 6 wks		

D-2

Appendix D: BW Agents - Vaccine, Therapeutics, and Prophylaxis (Continued)

DISEASE	VACCINE	CHEMOTHERAPY (Rx)	CHEMOPROPHYLAXIS (Px)	COMMENTS
Tularemia	IND - Live attenuated vaccine: single 0.1ml dose by scarification	Streptomycin 7.5-10 mg/kg IM bid x 10-14 d	Doxycycline 100 mg PO bid x 14 d	
		Gentamicin 3-5 mg/kg/d IV x 10-14 d	Tetracycline 500 mg PO qid x 14 d	
		Ciprofloxacin 400 mg IV q 12h until improved, then 500 mg PO q 12 h for total of 10 - 14 d	Ciprofloxacin 500 mg PO q 12 h for 14 d	
		Ciprofloxacin 750 mg PO q 12 h for 10 - 14 d		
Viral encephalitides	VEE DOD TC-83 live attenuated vaccine (IND): 0.5 mL SC x1 dose	Supportive therapy: analgesics and anticonvulsants prn	NA	TC-83 reactogenic in 20% No seroconversion in 20% Only effective against subtypes 1A, 1B, and 1C
	VEE DOD C-84 (formalin inactivated TC-83) (IND): 0.5 mL SC for up to 3 doses			C-84 vaccine used for non-responders to TC-83
	EEE inactivated (IND): 0.5 mL SC at 0 & 28 d			EEE and WEE inactivated vaccines are poorly
	WEE inactivated (IND): 0.5 mL SC at 0, 7, and 28 d			immunogenic. Multiple immunizations are required

Appendix D: BW Agents - Vaccine, Therapeutics, and Prophylaxis (Continued)

DISEASE	VACCINE	CHEMOTHERAPY (Rx)	CHEMOPROPHYLAXIS (Px)	COMMENTS
Viral Hemorrhagic Fevers	AHF Candid #1 vaccine (x-protection for BHF) (IND)	Ribavirin (CCHF/Lassa) (IND) 30 mg/kg IV initial dose; then 16 mg/kg IV q 6 h x 4 d; then 8 mg/kg IV q 8 h x 6 d	NA	Aggressive supportive care and management of hypotension very important
	RVF inactivated vaccine (IND)	Passive antibody for AHF, BHF, Lassa fever, and CCHF		
Smallpox	Wyeth calf lymph vaccinia vaccine (licensed): 1 dose by scarification	No current Rx other than supportive; Cidofovir (effective in vitro); animal studies ongoing	Vaccinia immune globulin 0.6 mL/kg IM (within 3 d of exposure, best within 24 h)	Pre and post exposure vaccination recommended if > 3 years since last vaccine
Botulism	DOD pentavalent toxoid for serotypes A - E (IND): 0.5 ml deep SC @ 0, 2 & 12 wk, then yearly boosters	DOD heptavalent equine despeciated antitoxin for serotypes A-G (IND): 1 vial (10 mL) IV	NA	Skin test for hypersensitivity before equine antitoxin administration
		CDC trivalent equine antitoxin for serotypes A, B, E (licensed)		
Staphylococcus Enterotoxin B	No vaccine available	Ventilatory support for inhalation exposure	NA	
Ricin	No vaccine available	Inhalation: supportive therapy G-I : gastric lavage, superactivated charcoal, cathartics	NA	
T-2 Mycotoxins	No vaccine available		Decontamination of clothing and skin	

Appendix E: Medical Sample Collection for Biological Threat Agents

This guide helps determine which clinical samples to collect from individuals exposed to aerosolized biological threat agents. Proper collection of specimens is dependent on the time-frame following exposure. Sample collection is described for "Early post-exposure", "Clinical", and "Convalescent/ Terminal/ Postmortem" time-frames. These time-frames are not rigid and will vary according to the concentration of the agent used, the agent strain, and predisposing health factors of the patient.

- Early post-exposure: when it is known that an individual has been exposed to a bioagent aerosol; aggressively attempt to obtain samples as indicated

- Clinical: samples from those individuals presenting with clinical symptoms

- Convalescent/Terminal/Postmortem: samples taken during convalescence, the terminal stages of infection or toxicosis or postmortem during autopsy

Shipping Samples: Most specimens sent rapidly (less than 24 h) to analytical labs require only blue or wet ice or refrigeration at 2 to 8 C. However, if the time span increases beyond 24 h, contact the USAMRIID "Hot-Line" (1-888-USA-RIID) for other shipping requirements such as shipment on dry-ice or in liquid nitrogen.

Blood samples: Several choices are offered based on availability of the blood collection tubes. Do not send blood in all the tubes listed, but merely choose one. Tiger-top tubes that have been centrifuged are preferred over red-top clot tubes with serum removed from the clot, but the latter will suffice. Blood culture bottles are also preferred over citrated blood for bacterial cultures.

Pathology samples: routinely include liver, lung, spleen, and regional or mesenteric lymph nodes. Additional samples requested are as follows: brain tissue for encephalomyelitis cases (mortality is rare) and the adrenal gland for Ebola (nice to have but not absolutely required).

Appendix E: Medical Sample Collection for Biological Threat Agents
Bacteria and Rickettsia

Early post-exposure	Clinical	Convalescent/ Terminal/Postmortem
Anthrax *Bacillus anthracis* <u>0 – 24 h</u> Nasal and throat swabs, induced respiratory secretions for culture, FA, and PCR	<u>24 to 72 h</u> Serum (TT, RT) for toxin assays Blood (E, C, H) for PCR. Blood (BC, C) for culture	<u>3 to 10 days</u> Serum (TT, RT) for toxin assays Blood (BC, C) for culture. Pathology samples
Plague *Yersinia pestis* <u>0 – 24 h</u> Nasal swabs, sputum, induced respiratory secretions for culture, FA, and PCR	<u>24 – 72 h</u> Blood (BC, C) and bloody sputum for culture and FA (C), F-1 Antigen assays (TT, RT), PCR (E, C, H)	<u>>6 days</u> Serum (TT, RT) for IgM later for IgG. Pathology samples
Tularemia *Francisella tularensis* <u>0 – 24 h</u> Nasal swabs, sputum, induced respiratory secretions for culture, FA and PCR	<u>24 – 72 h</u> Blood (BC, C) for culture Blood (E, C, H) for PCR Sputum for FA & PCR	<u>>6 days</u> Serum (TT, RT) for IgM and later IgG, agglutination titers. Pathology Samples
BC: Blood culture bottle C: Citrated blood (3-ml)	E: EDTA (3-ml) H: Heparin (3-ml)	TT: Tiger-top (5 – 10 ml) RT: Red top if no TT

E-3

Appendix E: Medical Sample Collection for Biological Threat Agents
Bacteria and Rickettsia

Early post-exposure	Clinical	Convalescent/ Terminal/Postmortem
Glanders *Burkholderia mallei* <u>0 – 24 h</u> Nasal swabs, sputum, induced respiratory secretions for culture and PCR.	<u>24 – 72 h</u> Blood (BC, C) for culture Blood (E, C, H) for PCR Sputum & drainage from skin lesions for PCR & culture.	<u>>6 days</u> Blood (BC, C) and tissues for culture. Serum (TT, RT) for immunoassays. Pathology samples.
Brucellosis *Brucella abortus, suis*, & *melitensis* <u>0 – 24 h</u> Nasal swabs, sputum, induced respiratory secretions for culture and PCR.	<u>24 – 72 h</u> Blood (BC, C) for culture. Blood (E, C, H) for PCR.	<u>>6 days</u> Blood (BC, C) and tissues for culture. Serum (TT, RT) for immunoassays. Pathology samples
Q-Fever *Coxiella burnetii* <u>0 – 24 h</u> Nasal swabs, sputum, induced respiratory secretions for culture and PCR.	<u>2 to 5 days</u> Blood (BC, C) for culture in eggs or mouse inoculation Blood (E, C, H) for PCR.	<u>>6 days</u> Blood (BC, C) for culture in eggs or mouse inoculation Pathology samples.
BC: Blood culture bottle C: Citrated blood (3-ml)	E: EDTA (3-ml) H: Heparin (3-ml)	TT: Tiger-top (5 - 10 ml) RT: Red top if no TT

Appendix E: Medical Sample Collection for Biological Threat Agents
Toxins

Early post-exposure	Clinical	Convalescent/ Terminal/Postmortem
Botulism Botulinum toxin from *Clostridium botulinum* <u>0 – 24 h</u> Nasal swabs, induced respiratory secretions for PCR (contaminating bacterial DNA) and toxin assays. Serum (TT, RT) for toxin assays	<u>24 to 72 h</u> Nasal swabs, respiratory secretions for PCR (contaminating bacterial DNA) and toxin assays.	<u>>6 days</u> Usually no IgM or IgG Pathology samples (liver and spleen for toxin detection)
Ricin Intoxication Ricin toxin from Castor beans <u>0 – 24 h</u> Nasal swabs, induced respiratory secretions for PCR (contaminating castor bean DNA) and toxin assays. Serum (TT) for toxin assays	<u>36 to 48 h</u> Serum (TT, RT) for toxin assay Tissues for immunohisto-logical stain in pathology samples.	<u>>6 days</u> Serum (TT, RT) for IgM and IgG in survivors
Staph enterotoxicosis *Staphylococcus* Enterotoxin B <u>0 – 3 h</u> Nasal swabs, induced respiratory secretions for PCR (contaminating bacterial DNA) and toxin assays. Serum (TT, RT) for toxin assays	<u>2 - 6 h</u> Urine for immunoassays Nasal swabs, induced respiratory secretions for PCR (contaminating bacterial DNA) and toxin assays. Serum (TT, RT) for toxin assays	<u>>6 days</u> Serum for IgM and IgG
T-2 toxicosis <u>0 – 24 h postexposure</u> Nasal & throat swabs, induced respiratory secretions for immunoassays, HPLC/ mass spectrometry (HPLC/MS).	<u>1 to 5 days</u> Serum (TT, RT), tissue for toxin detection	<u>>6 days postexposure</u> Urine for detection of toxin metabolites
BC: Blood culture bottle C: Citrated blood (3-ml)	E: EDTA (3-ml) H: Heparin (3-ml)	TT: Tiger-top (5 - 10 ml) RT: Red top if no TT

E-5

Appendix E: Medical Sample Collection for Biological Threat Agents
Viruses

Early post-exposure	Clinical	Convalescent/ Terminal/Postmortem
Equine Encephalmyelitis VEE, EEE and WEE viruses <u>0 – 24 h</u> Nasal swabs & induced respiratory secretions for RT-PCR and viral culture	<u>24 to 72 h</u> Serum & Throat swabs for culture (TT, RT), RT-PCR (E, C, H, TT, RT) and Antigen ELISA (TT, RT), CSF, Throat swabs up to 5 days	<u>>6 days</u> Serum (TT, RT) for IgM Pathology samples plus brain
Ebola <u>0 – 24 h</u> Nasal swabs & induced respiratory secretions for RT-PCR and viral culture	<u>2 to 5 days</u> Serum (TT, RT) for viral culture	<u>>6 days</u> Serum (TT, RT) for viral culture. Pathology samples plus adrenal gland.
Pox (Small pox, monkey pox) *Orthopoxvirus* <u>0 – 24 h</u> Nasal swabs & induced respiratory secretions for PCR and viral culture	<u>2 to 5 days</u> Serum (TT, RT) for viral culture	<u>>6 days</u> Serum (TT, RT) for viral culture. Drainage from skin lesions/ scrapings for microscopy, EM, viral culture, PCR. Pathology samples
BC: Blood culture bottle C: Citrated blood (3-ml)	E: EDTA (3-ml)H: Heparin (3-ml)	TT: Tiger-top (5 - 10 ml) RT: Red top if no TT

E-6

Appendix F: Specimens for Laboratory Diagnosis

Agent	Face or Nasal Swab[1]	Blood Culture	Smear	Acute & Convalescent Sera	Stool	Urine	Other
Anthrax	+	+	Pleural and CS fluids mediastinal lymph node spleen	+	+	-	Cut. Lesion aspirates
Brucellosis	+	+	-	+	-	-	Bone marrow and spinal fluid cultures; tissues, exudates
Cholera	-	-	-	+	+	-	
Plague	+	+	Sputum	+	-	-	Bubo aspirate, CSF, sputum, lesion scraping, LN aspirate
Tularemia	+	+	+[2]	+	-	-	
Q-fever	+	[4]	Lesions	+	-	-	Lung, spleen, lymph nodes, bone marrow
Congo-Crimean Hemorrhagic Fever	+	[3]	-	+	-	-	Liver
VEE	+	[3]	-	+	-	-	CSF
Clostridial Toxins	+	-	Wound tissues	+	+	-	
SEB Toxin	+	-	-	+	+	+	Lung, kidney
Ricin Toxin	+	-	-	+	+	+	Spleen, lung, kidney

[1] Within 18-24 hours
[2] Fluorescent antibody test on infected lymph node smears. Gram stain has little value.
[3] Virus isolation from blood or throat swabs in appropriate containment.
[4] *C. burnetii* can persist for days in blood and resists desiccation. EDTA anticoagulated blood preferred. Culturing should not be done except in BL3 containment.

F-1

Appendix G: BW Agent Lab Identification

Agent	Gold Standard	Antigen Detection	IgG	IgM	PCR	Animals
		Immunoassays				
Aflatoxins	Mass spectrometry					
Arboviruses (incl. alphaviruses)	Virus isolation/FA, neutralization	X	X	X	X	X
Bacillus anthracis	FA/Std. Microbiology	X (PA)	X	X	X	X
Bacillus globigii	Std. Microbiology				X	
Bacillus thuringiensis	Std. Microbiology				X	
Bot Toxins (A-G)/*C. botulinum*	Mouse neutralization/ standard microbiology	X (A,B,E Toxin)			X	X
Brucella sp.	FA/Std. Microbiology	X	X	X	X	X
C. burnetii	FA/eggs or cell Cx/serology	X	X	X	X	X
C. perfringens/toxins	Std. Micro./ELISA (alpha and enterotoxin	X	X		X	
F. tularensis	FA/Std. Microbiology	X	X	X	X	X
Filoviruses	Virus isolation/neutralization	X	X	X	X	X
Hantaviruses	Virus isolation/ FA/neutralization	X	X	X	X	X
Orthopox Viruses	Virus isolation/ FA/neutralization	X	X		X	X
Ricin Toxin	ELISA	X	X	X	X	X
Saxitoxin	Bioassay		(neutralizing antibodies)			X
SEA Toxin	ELISA	X	X		*	
SEB Toxin	ELISA	X	X		*	X
Shigella sp.	Std. Microbiology	X			X	
Tetrodotoxins	Bioassay	X	(neutralizing antibodies)			X

G-1

Appendix G: BW Agent Lab Identification (Continued)

Agent	Gold Standard	Antigen Detection	IgG	IgM	PCR	Animals
Vibrio cholerae	Std. Microbiology/serology	X(toxin)	X	X	X	
Yersinia pestis	FA/Std. Microbiology	X (F1)	X	X	X	X

*Toxin gene detected
ELISA - enzyme-linked immunosorbent assays
FA - indirect or direct immunofluorescence assays
Std. Micro./serology - standard microbiological techniques available, including electron microscopy

Appendix H: Differential Diagnosis of Chemical Nerve Agent, Botulinum Toxin and SEB Intoxication Following Inhalation Exposure

	Chemical Nerve Agent	Botulinum Toxin	SEB
Time to Symptoms	Minutes	Hours (12-48)	Hours (1-6)
Nervous	Convulsions, Muscle twitching	Progressive paralysis	Headache, Muscle aches
Cardiovascular	Slow heart rate	Normal rate	Normal or rapid heart rate
Respiratory	Difficult breathing, airway constriction	Normal, then progressive paralysis	Nonproductive cough; Severe cases; chest pain/difficult breathing
Gastrointestinal	Increased motility, pain, diarrhea	Decreased motility	Nausea, vomiting and/or diarrhea
Ocular	Small pupils	Droopy eyelids, Large pupils	May see "red eyes" (conjuntival infection)
Salivary	Profuse, watery saliva	Normal; difficulty swallowing	May be slightly increased quantities of saliva
Death	Minutes	2-3 days	Unlikely
Response to Atropine/2PAM-CL	Yes	No	Atropine may reduce gastrointestinal symptoms

Appendix I: Comparative Lethality of Selected Toxins & Chemical Agents in Laboratory Mice

AGENT	LD$_{50}$ (µg/kg)	MOLECULAR WEIGHT	SOURCE
Botulinum toxin	0.001	150,000	Bacterium
Shiga toxin	0.002	55,000	Bacterium
Tetanus toxin	0.002	150,000	Bacterium
Abrin	0.04	65,000	Plant (Rosary Pea)
Diphtheria toxin	0.10	62,000	Bacterium
Maitotoxin	0.10	3,400	Marine Dinoflagellate
Palytoxin	0.15	2,700	Marine Soft Coral
Ciguatoxin	0.40	1,000	Marine Dinoflagellate
Textilotoxin	0.60	80,000	Elapid Snake
C. perfringens toxins	0.1 – 5.0	35-40,000	Bacterium
Batrachotoxin	2.0	539	Arrow-Poison Frog
Ricin	3.0	64,000	Plant (Castor Bean)
alpha-Conotoxin	5.0	1,500	Cone Snail
Taipoxin	5.0	46,000	Elapid Snake
Tetrodotoxin	8.0	319	Puffer Fish
alpha-Tityustoxin	9.0	8,000	Scorpion
Saxitoxin	10.0 (Inhal 2.0)	299	Marine Dinoflagellate
VX	15.0	267	Chemical Agent
SEB (Rhesus/Aerosol)	27.0 (ED$_{50}$~pg)	28,494	Bacterium
Anatoxin-A(s)	50.0	500	Blue-Green Algae
Microcystin	50.0	994	Blue-Green Algae
Soman (GD)	64.0	182	Chemical Agent
Sarin (GB)	100.0	140	Chemical Agent
Aconitine	100.0	647	Plant (Monkshood)
T-2 Toxin	1,210.0	466	Fungal Myotoxin

Appendix J. Aerosol Toxicity in LD_{50} vs. Quantity of Toxin

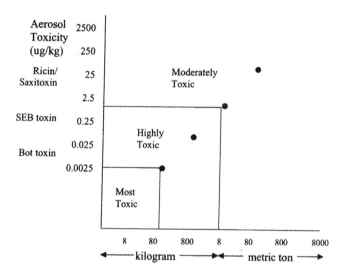

Aerosol toxicity in LD_{50} (see Appendix C) vs. quantity of toxin required to provide a theoretically effective open-air exposure, under ideal meteorological conditions, to an area 100 km^2. Ricin, saxitoxin and botulinum toxins kill at the concentrations depicted. (Patrick and Spertzel, 1992: Based on Cader K.L., BWL Tech Study #3, Mathematical models for dosage and casualty resulting from single point and line source release of aerosol near ground level, DTIC#AD3 10-361, Dec 1957)

Appendix K: References and Emergency Response Contacts

Journals with Biological Weapon Theme issues:

Annals of Emergency Medicine-August 1999
Emerging Infectious Diseases-July/August 1999
Journal of the American Medical Association-August 6, 1997
Journal of Public Health Management and Practice-July 2000

Background/Overview

Cieslak TJ, Eitzen EM. Bioterrorism: Agents of concern. J Public Health Management Practice 2000;6:19-29

Cieslak TJ, Christopher GW, Kortepeter MG, Rowe JR, Pavlin JA, Culpepper RC, Eitzen EM. Immunization against potential biological warfare agents. Clin Infect Dis 2000 [in press].

Henretig FM, Cieslak TJ, Madsen JM, Eitzen EM, Flesiher GR. The emergency department response to incidents of chemical and biological terrorism. In: Textbook of Pediatric Emergency Medicine, Fleisher GR, Ludwig S, eds. Lippincott, Williams, and Wilkins, Philadelphia, 2000, pp. 1763-84.

Kortepeter MG, Parker GW. Potential Biological Weapons Threats. Emerging Infectious Diseases 2000; 5(4): 523-527.

Macintyre AG, Christopher GW, Eitzen EM Jr., Gum R, Weir S, DeAtley C, Tonat K, Barbera JA. Weapons of mass destruction events with contaminated casualties: effective planning for health care facilities. *JAMA* 2000:283;242-249.

McGovern TW, Christopher GW, Eitzen EM Jr. Cutaneous manifestations of biological warfare and related threat agents. *Arch Dermatol*;1999:135:311-322.

Books:

Biological Weapons: Limiting the Threat. Lederberg J (ed.). Cambridge,Mass;The MIT Press:1999.

Institute of Medicine and National Research Council. *Chemical and Biological Terrorism. Research and Development to Improve Civilian Medical Response*. Washington, D.C.; National Academy Press;1999.

Ali J, Dwyer A, Eldridge J, Lewis FA, Patrick WC, Sidell, FR. *Jane's Chemical-Biological Defense Guidebook*. Alexandria, Va; Jane's Information Group; 1999.

Alibek K, with Handelman S. *Biohazard*. New York; Random House; 1999

Benenson, AS. Control of Communicable Diseases Manual (16th ed.) American Public Health Association, Baltimore: United Book Press Co; 1995.

Falkenrath RA, Newman RD, Thayer BA. *America's Achilles' Heel. Nuclear, Biological, and Chemical Terrorism and Covert Attack.* Cambridge, Mass; The MIT Press, 1998.

Fenner F, Henderson DA, Arita I, Jezek Z, Ladnyi ID. Smallpox and its Eradication. Geneva, Switzerland: World Health Organization;1988.

Fields Virology (3d ed.), Fields BN, Knipe DM, Howley PM, et al (eds). Philadelphia: Lippincott-Raven; 1996.

Guillemin J. Anthrax. 1999

Hunter's Tropical Medicine (8th ed.). G. Thomas Strickland, (ed.). 2000: W.B. Saunders Co., Philadelphia.

Medical aspects of chemical and biological warfare. (TMM series. Part I, Warfare, weaponry, and the casualty). Sidell FR, Takafuji ET, Franz DR (eds.). Office of The Surgeon General at TMM Publications, Borden Institute, Washington, D.C., 1997.

K-3

Medical Management of Biological Casualties Handbook (3rd ed.). Eitzen E, Pavlin J, Cieslak T, Christopher G, Culpepper R (eds.).Fort Detrick, Frederick, MD: U.S. Army Medical Research Institute of Infectious Diseases; 1998.

Principles and Practice of Infectious Diseases (5th ed.). Mandell GL, Bennett JE, Dolin R. 2000: Churchill Livingstone, Philadelphia.

Regis E. *The Biology of Doom*. New York; Henry Holt and Co.; 1999.

Web Sources

Biolectures:
www.nbc-med.org/SiteContent/MedRef/OnlineRef/GovDocs/BioWarfare

www.nbc-med.org/SiteContent/MedRef/OnlineRef/GovDocs/Anthrax

www.nbc-med.org/SiteContent/MedRef/OnlineRef/GovDocs/BioAgents.html

www.nbc-med.org/SiteContent/MedRef/OnlineRef/GovDocs/SmallPox/index.htm

www.nbc-med.org/SiteContent/MedRef/OnlineRef/GovDocs/Viral/index.htm

www.nbc-med.org. US Army Surgeon General's site on nuclear, biological, chemical defense.

www.usamriid.army.mil. USAMRIID website

www.apic.org. Association of Professionals in Infection Control and Epidemiology. Contains bioterrorism response plan

www.hopkins-biodefense.org Johns Hopkins University Center for Civilian Biodefense

www.anthrax.osd.mil Anthrax Vaccine Implementation Program

www.bt.cdc.gov CDC's bioterrorism preparedness and response website

Journal Articles:

Anthrax
Abramova, F.A., Grinberg, L.M., Yampolskaya, O.V., Walker, D.H., *Pathology of Inhalational Anthrax in 42 Cases from the Sverdlovsk Outbreak of 1979*. Proceedings of the National Academy of Sciences, USA (1993), 90:2291-4.

Centers for Disease Control and Prevention. *Bioterrorism Alleging Use of Anthrax and Interim Guidelines for Management-United States, 1998*. Morbidity and Mortality Weekly Report (1999), 48:69-74.

Cieslak TJ, Eitzen EM. Clinical and epidemiologic principles of anthrax. Emerging Infect Dis 1999;5:-5.

Dixon TC, Meselson M, Guillemin J, Hanna PC. Anthrax. *New Engl J Med* 1999;341:815-826.

Friedlander AM, Welkos SLL, Pitt MLM, et al. Postexposure prophylaxis against experimental inhalation anthrax. *J Infect Dis* 1993;167:1239-42.

Jackson, P.J., Hugh-Jones, M.E., Adair, D.M., et al. *Polymerase Chain Reaction Analysis of Tissue Samples from the 1979 Sverdlovsk Anthrax Victims: The Presence of Multiple Bacillus Anthracis Strains in Different Victims*. Proceedings of the National Academy of Sciences, USA (1998), 95:1224-9.

Garner, J.S., *Hospital Infection Control Practices Advisory Committee. Guidelines for Isolation Precautions in Hospitals*. Infectious Control Hospital, Epidemiology (1996), 17:53-80, and American Journal of Infection Control (1996), 24:24-52

Meselson M, Guillemin JG, Hugh-Jones M, et al. The Sverdlovsk anthrax outbreak of 1979. *Science*;1994:266:1202-1207.

Pile JC, Malone JD, Eitzen EM, Friedlander AM. Anthrax as a potential biological warfare agent. *Arch Intern Med* 1998;158:429-34.

Pomerantsev, A.P., Staritsin, N.A., Mockov, Y.V., Marinin, L.I., *Expression of Cereolysine AB Genes in Bacillus anthracis Vaccine Strain Ensures Protection Against Experimental Hemolytic Anthrax Infection.* Vaccine (1997), 15:1846-1850.

Brucellosis
Mousa ARM, Elhag KM, Khogali M, Marafie AA. The nature of human brucellosis in Kuwait: study of 379 cases. Rev Infect Dis 1988;10:211-7.

Young EJ. An overview of human brucellosis. Clin Infect Dis 1995;21:283-90

Glanders/Melioidosis
CDC. Laboratory-acquired human glanders - Marlyland, May 2000. MMWR 2000;49:532-535.

Chaowagul W, Suputtamongkol Y, Dance DAB, et al. Relapse in Melioidosis: incidence and risk factors. J Infect Dis. 1993;168:1181-5.

Howe C, Miller WR. Human Glanders: report of six cases Ann Int Med 1947; 26: 93-115.

Leelarasamee A, Bovornkitti S. Melioidosis: review and update. Rev Infect Dis. 1989;11(3): 413-23.

Misra VC, Mukesh S, Thakur V. Glanders: an appraisal and its control in India. Indian Veterinary Medical Journal 1995;19(2):87-98.

Plague

Byrne, WR, Welkos, SL, Pitt, ML, et.al. Antibiotic Treatment of Experimental Pneumonic Plague in Mice. *Antimicrobial Agents and Chemotherapy.* 1998;42:675-681.

CDC. Prevention of Plague: Recommendations of the Advisory Committee on Immunization Practices (ACIP). *MMWR* 1996;45:1-15.

Heath, DG, Anderson, GW, Mauro, JM, et.al. Protection Against Experimental Bubonic and Pneumonic Plague by a Recombinant Capsular F1-V Antigen Fusion Protein Vaccine. *Vaccine* 1998;16:1131-1137.

Inglesby, TV, Dennis, DT, Henderson, DA, et.al. Plague as a Biological Weapon: Medical and Public Health Management. *JAMA* 2000;283:2281-2290.

Perry, RD and Fetherson, JD Yersinia pestis—Etiologic Agent of Plague. *Clinical Microbiol Reviews* 1997;10:35-66.

Smallpox

Barquet N, Domingo P. Smallpox: The triumph over the most terrible of the ministers of death. Ann Intern Med 1997;127;635-642.

Breman JG, Henderson DA. Poxvirus dilemmas-monkeypox, smallpox, and biologic terrorism. N Engl J Med 1998;339:556-9.

CDC. Human monkeypox-Kasai Oriental, Zaire, 1996-1997. MMWR 1997;46:301-7.

CDC. Human Monkeypox-Kasai Oriental, Democratic Republic of Congo, February 1996-October 1997. MMWR 1997;46:1168-71.

CDC. *Vaccinia (Smallpox) Vaccine: Recommendations of the ACIP.* Morbidity and Mortality Weekly Report (1991), 40:RR-14 (Suppl).

Disseminated vaccinia in a military recruit with human immunodeficiency virus (HIV) disease. N Engl J Med 1987;316:673-6.

Henderson DA. Edward Jenner's vaccine. Publ Health Rep 1997;112:117-121.

Henderson DA, Inglesby TV, Bartlett JG, et al. Smallpox as a biological weapon. Medical and Public Health Management. JAMA 1999;281:2127-2137.

Kesson A, Ferguson JK, Rawlinson WD, Cunningham AL. Progressive vaccinia treated with ribavirin and vacinia immune globulin. Clin Infect Dis 1997;25:911-4

McClain DJ, Harrison S, Yeager CL, et al. Immunologic responses to vaccinia vaccines administered by different parenteral routes. J Infect Dis 1997;175:756-63

Radetsky M. Smallpox: a history of its rise and fall. Pediatr Infect Dis J 1999;18:85-93.

Vaccinia (smallpox) vaccine: recommendations of the Immunization Practices +Advisory Committee (ACIP). MMWR 1991;40:RR-14 (Suppl)

Viral Hemorrhagic Fevers
Armstrong LR, Dembry LM, Rainey PM, Russi MB, et al. Management of a Sabia virus-infected patient in a US Hospital. Infect Control Hosp Epidemiol 1999;20:176-82.

Barry M, Russi M, Armstrong L, et al. Brief report: treatment of a laboratory acquired Sabia virus infection. N Engl J Med 1995;333:294-6.

CDC. Management of patients with suspected viral hemorrhagic fever. MMWR 1988;37: S-3 (Suppl).

CDC. Update: Management of patients with suspected viral hemorrhagic fever-United States. MMWR 1995;44:475-9.

CDC. Ebola virus infection in imported primates-Virginia, 1989. MMWR 1989;38:831-9.

CDC. Update: Filovirus infections among persons with occupational exposure to nonhuman primates. MMWR 1990;39:266-7.

Christopher GW, Eitzen EM Jr. Air evacuation under high-level biosafety containment: the Aeromedical Isolation Team. *Emerg Infect Dis* 1999;241-246. Available from: URL http: // www. cdc. gov/ncidod/EID/vol5no2/ christopher.htm

Clausen L, Bothwell TH, Isaacson M, et al. Isolation and handling of patients with dangerous infectious disease. S Afr Med J 1978;53:238-42.

Dalgard DW, Hardy, RJ, Pearson SL, et al. Combined simian hemorrhagic fever and ebola virus infection in cynomolgus monkeys. Lab Anim Sci 1992;42:152-7.

Fisher-Hoch SP, Price ME, Craven RB, et al. Safe intensive-care management of a severe case of Lassa fever with simple barrier nursing techniques. Lancet 1985;2:1227-9.

Hill EE, McKee KT. Isolation and biocontainment of patients with highly hazardous infectious diseases. J US Army Med Dept 1991;PB 8-91-1/2:10-4.

Holmes GP, McCormick JB, Trock SC, et al. Lassa fever In the United States: investigation of a case and new guidelines for management. N Enl J Med 1990;323:1120-3.

Jahrling PB, Geisbert TW, Dalgard DW, et al. Preliminary report: isolation of Ebola virus from monkeys imported to USA. Lancet 1990;335:502-5.

Johnson KM, Monath TP. Imported Lassa fever-reexamining the algorithms. New Engl J Med 1990;323:1139-40.

Peters CJ, Sanchez A, Rollin PE, Ksiazek TG, Murphy FA. Filoviridae: Marburg and Ebola viruses. pp 1161-76, *Fields Virology* (3d ed.), Fields BN, Knipe DM, Howley PM, et al (eds). Philadelphia: Lippincott-Raven; 1996.

Trexler PC, RTD Emond, Evans B. Negative-pressure plastic isolator for patients with dangerous infections. Brit Med J 1977; 559-61.

Wilson KE, Driscoll DM. Mobile high-containment isolation: a unique patient care modality. Am J Infect Cont 1987;15:120-4.

Toxins
Burrows, WD and Renner, SE. Biological Warfare Agents as Threats to Potable Water. *Environmental Health Perspectives*, 1999;107:975-984.

Franz, DR. Defense Against Toxin Weapons. 1997 Medical Research and Materiel Command, pp. 1-49.

Franz, DR, Pitt, LM, Clayton, MA, et.al. Efficacy of Prophylactic and Therapeutic Administration of Antitoxin for Inhalation Botulism. *Botulinum and Tetanus Neurotoxins* [Proc. Int. Conf.] 1993;473-6.

Goldfrank, LR and Flomenbaum, NE. Botulism, in Goldfrank's Toxicologic Emergencies, 6th ed. Stamford, CT: Appleton and Lange, 1177-1189.

Parker, DT, Parker, AC, Ramachandran, CK. Joint CB Technical Data Source Book, Volume VI. Toxin Agents, Part 3, Ricin. 1996 DPG/JCP-96/007.

Patrick, WC. Analysis of Botulinum Toxin, Type A, as a Biological Warfare Threat. May 1998, pp.1-26 (unpublished monograph).

Rutala, WA and Weber, DJ. Uses of Inorganic Hypochlorite (Bleach) in Health-Care Facilities. *Clinical Microbiology Reviews*, 1997;10:597-610.

Federal Bureau of Investigation (FBI) Field Offices

Revised FBI 1/5/99

FIELD OFFICE	STREET ADDRESS	ZIP CODE	TELEPHONE No.
Albany, NY	200 McCarty Avenue	12209	518/465-7551
Albuquerque, NM	415 Silver Avenue, SW, Suite 300	87102	505/224-2000
Anchorage, AK	101 East 6th Avenue	99501	907/258-5322
Atlanta, GA	2635 Century Parkway, NE; Suite 400	30345	404/679-9000
Baltimore, MD	7142 Ambassador Road	21244	410/265-8080
Birmingham, AL	2121 8th Avenue, N., Room 1400	35203	205/326-6166
Boston, MA	One Center Plaza, Suite 600	02108	617/742-5533
Buffalo, NY	One FBI Plaza	14202	716-856-7800
Charlotte, NC	400 S. Tryon Street, Suite 900 Wachovia Blvd	28285	704/377-9200
Chicago, IL	219 S. Dearborn Street, Room 905	60604	312/431-1333
Cincinnati, OH	550 Main Street, Room 9000	45202	513/421-4310
Cleveland, OH	1240 East 9th Street, Room 3005	44199	216/522-1400
Columbia, SC	151 Westpark Blvd.	29210	803/551-1200
Dallas, TX	1801 N. Lamar, Suite 300	75202	214/720-2200
Denver, CO	1961 Stout Street, Room 1823, FOB	80294	303/629-7171
Detroit, MI	477 Michigan Avenue, P.V. McNamara FOB, 26th Floor	48226	313/965-2323
El Paso, TX	Suite 3000, 660 South Mesa Hills Drive	79912	915/832-5000
Honolulu, HI	300 Ala Moana Blvd., Room 4-230, Kalanianaole FOB	96850	808/521-1411
Houston, TX	2500 East T.C. Jester	77008	713/693-5000
Indianapolis, IN	575 N. Pennsylvania St., Room 679, FOB	46204	317/639-3301
Jackson, MS	100 W. Capitol Street, Suite 1553, FOB	39269	601/948-5000
Jacksonville, FL	7820 Arlington Expy, Suite 200	32211	904/721-1211
Kansas City, MO	1300 Summit Street	64105	816/221-6100
Knoxville, TN	710 Locust Street, Suite 600	37902	423/544-0751
Las Vegas, NV	John Lawrence Bailey Bldg., 700 E. Charleston Blvd.	89104	702/385-1281
Little Rock, AR	10825 Financial Centre Pkwy., Suite 200	72211	501/221-9100
Los Angeles, CA	11000 Wilshire Blvd., Suite 1700 FOB	90024	310/477-6565
Louisville, KY	600 Martin Luther King Jr. Pl., Room 500	40202	502/583-3941
Memphis, TN	225 North Humphreys Blvd., Suite 3000, Eagle Crest Bldg.	38120	901/747-4300

K-14

Federal Bureau of Investigation (FBI) Field Offices (Continued)

FIELD OFFICE	STREET ADDRESS	ZIP CODE	TELEPHONE No.
Miami, FL	16320 NW 2nd Avenue, N. Miami Beach	33169	305/944-9101
Milwaukee, WI	330 E. Kilbourn Avenue, Suite 600	53202	414/276-4684
Minneapolis, MN	111 Washington Avenue South, Suite 1100	55401	612/376-3200
Mobile, AL	One St. Louis Street, 3rd Floor, One St. Louis Centre	36602	334/438-3674
New Haven, CT	150 Court Street, Room 535 FOB	06510	203/777-6311
New Orleans, LA	1250 Poydras Street, Suite 2200	70113	504/522-4671
New York City, NY	26 Federal Plaza, 23rd Floor	10278	212/384-1000
Newark, NJ	One Gateway Center, 22nd Floor	07102	973/622-5613
Norfolk, VA	150 Corporate Blvd.	23502	757/455-0100
Oklahoma City, OK	50 Penn Place, Suite 1600	73118	405/290-7770
Omaha, NE	10755 Burt Street	68114	402/493-8688
Philadelphia, PA	600 Arch Street, 8th Floor; William J. Green, Jr., FOB	19106	215/418-4000
Phoenix, AZ	201 E. Indianola Avenue, Suite 400	85012	602/279-5511
Pittsburgh, PA	700 Grant Street, Suite 300 USPO	15219	412/471-2000
Portland, OR	1500 S.W. 1st Avenue, Suite 400; Crown Plaza Bldg.	97201	503/224-4181
Richmond, VA	111 Greencourt Road	23228	804/261-1044
Sacramento, CA	4500 Orange Grove Avenue	95841	916/481-9110
Salt Lake City, UT	257 East 200 South, Suite 1200	84111	801/579-1400
San Antonio. TX	615 E. Houston Street, Suite 200; US Post Office & Courthouse Bldg.	78205	210/225-6741
San Diego, CA	9797 Aero Drive	92123	619/565-1255
San Francisco, CA	450 Golden Gate Avenue, 13th Floor	94102	415/553-7400
San Juan, PR	150 Carlos Chardon, Room 526; U.S. Federal Building, Hato Roy, PR	00918	787/754-6000
Seattle, WA	915 Second Avenue, Room 710	98174	206/622-0460
Springfield, IL	400 W. Monroe Street, Suite 400	62704	217/522-9675
St. Louis, Mo	2222 Market Street	63103	314/231-4324
Tampa, FL	500 E. Zack Street, Suite 610 FOB	33602	813/273-4566
Washington, D.C.	601 4th Street, NW	20535	202/278-2000

K-15

Telephone Directory of State and Territorial Public Health Directors

Alabama
Alabama Department of Public Health
State Health Officer
Phone No. (334) 206-5200
Fax No. (334) 206-2008

Alaska
Division of Public Health
Alaska Department of Health and Social Services
Director
Phone No. (907) 465-3090
Fax No. (907) 586-1877

American Samoa
Department of Health
American Samoa Government
Director
Phone No. (684) 633-4606
Fax No. (684) 633-5379

Arizona
Arizona Department of Health Services
Director
Phone No. (602) 542-1025
Fax No. (602) 542-1062

Arkansas
Arkansas Department of Health
Director
Phone No. (501) 661-2417
Fax No. (501) 671-1450

California
California Department of Health Services
State Health Officer
Phone No. (916) 657-1493
Fax No. (916) 657-3089

Colorado
Colorado Department of Public Health & Environment
Executive Director
Phone No. (303) 692-2011
Fax No. (303) 691-7702

Connecticut
Connecticut Department of Public Health
Commissioner
Phone No. (860) 509-7101
Fax No. (860) 509-7111

Delaware
Division of Public Health
Delaware Department of Health and Social Services
Director
Phone No. (302) 739-4700
Fax No. (302) 739-6659

K-17

District of Columbia
DC Department of Health
Acting Director
Phone No. (202) 645-5556
Fax No. (202) 645-0526

Florida
Florida Department of Health
Secretary and State Health Officer
Phone No. (850) 487-2945
Fax No. (850) 487-3729

Georgia
Division of Public Health
Georgia Department of Human Resources
Director
Phone No. (404) 657-2700
Fax No. (404) 657-2715

Guam
Department of Public Health & Social Services
Government of Guam
Director of Health
Phone No. (671) 735-7102
Fax No. (671) 734-5910

Hawaii
Hawaii Department of Health
Director
Phone No. (808) 586-4410
Fax No. (808) 586-4444

K-18

Idaho
Division of Health
Idaho Department of Health and Welfare
Administrator
Phone No. (208) 334-5945
Fax No. (208) 334-6581

Illinois
Illinois Department of Public Health
Director of Public Health
Phone No. (217) 782-4977
Fax No. (217) 782-3987

Indiana
Indiana State Department of Health
State Health Commissioner
Phone No. (317) 233-7400
Fax No. (317) 233-7387

Iowa
Iowa Department of Public Health
Director of Public Health
Phone No. (515) 281-5605
Fax No. (515) 281-4958

Kansas
Kansas Department of Health and Environment
Director of Health
Phone No. (785) 296-1343
Fax No. (785) 296-1562

Kentucky
Kentucky Department for Public Health
Commissioner
Phone No. (502) 564-3970
Fax No. (502) 564-6533

Louisiana
Louisiana Department of Health and Hospitals
Asst Secretary and State Health Officer
Phone No. (504) 342-8093
Fax No. (504) 342-8098

Maine
Maine Bureau of Health
Maine Department of Human Services
Director
Phone No. (207) 287-3201
Fax No. (207) 287-4631

Mariana Islands
Department of Public Health & Environmental Services
Commonwealth of the Northern Mariana Islands
Secretary of Health and Environmental Services
Phone No. (670) 234-8950
Fax No. (670) 234-8930

Marshall Islands
Republic of the Marshall Islands
Majuro Hospital
Minister of Health & Environmental Services
Phone No. (692) 625-3355
Fax No. (692) 625-3432

K-20

Maryland
Maryland Dept of Health and Mental Hygiene
Secretary
Phone No. (410) 767-6505
Fax No. (410) 767-6489

Massachusetts
Massachusetts Department of Public Health
Commissioner
Phone No. (617) 624-5200
Fax No. (617) 624-5206

Michigan
Michigan Depart of Community Health
Chief Executive and Medical Officer
Phone No. (517) 335-8024
Fax No. (517) 335-9476

Micronesia
Department of Health Services
FSM National Government
Secretary of Health
Phone No. (691) 320-2619
Fax No. (691) 320-5263

Minnesota
Minnesota Department of Health
Commissioner of Health
Phone No. (651) 296-8401
Fax No. (651) 215-5801

Mississippi
Mississippi State Department of Health
State Health Officer and Chief Executive
Phone No. (601) 960-7634
Fax No. (601) 960-7931

Missouri
Missouri Department of Health
Director
Phone No. (573) 751-6001
Fax No. (573) 751-6041

Montana
Montana Dept of Public Health & Human Services,
Director
Phone No. (406) 444-5622
Fax No. (406) 444-1970

Nebraska
Nebraska Health and Human Services System
Chief Medical Officer
Phone No. (402) 471-8399
Fax No. (402) 471-9449

Nevada
Division of Health
NV State Dept of Human Resources
State Health Officer
Phone No. (702) 687-3786
Fax No. (702) 687-3859

K-22

New Hampshire
New Hampshire Department of Health & Human
Services
Medical Director
Phone No. (603) 271-4372
Fax No. (603) 271-4827

New Jersey
New Jersey Department of Health & Senior Services
Commissioner of Health
Phone No. (609) 292-7837
Fax No. (609) 292-0053

New Mexico
New Mexico Department of Health
Secretary
Phone No. (505) 827-2613
Fax No. (505) 827-2530

New York
New York State Department of Health
ESP-Corning Tower, 14th Floor
Albany, NY 12237
Commissioner of Health
Phone No. (518) 474-2011
Fax No. (518) 474-5450

North Carolina
NC Dept of Health and Human Services
State Health Director
Phone No. (919) 733-4392
Fax No. (919) 715-4645

North Dakota
North Dakota Department of Health
State Health Officer
Phone No. (701) 328-2372
Fax No. (701) 328-4727

Ohio
Ohio Department of Health
Director of Health
Phone No. (614) 466-2253
Fax No. (614) 644-0085

Oklahoma
Oklahoma State Department of Health
Commissioner of Health
Phone No. (405) 271-4200
Fax No. (405) 271-3431

Oregon
Oregon Health Division
Oregon Dept of Human Resources
Administrator
Phone No. (503) 731-4000
Fax No. (503) 731-4078

Palau, Republic of
Ministry of Health, Republic of Palau
Minister of Health
Phone No. (680) 488-2813
Fax No. (680) 488-1211

Pennsylvania
Pennsylvania Department of Health
Secretary of Health
Phone No. (717) 787-6436
Fax No. (717) 787-0191

Puerto Rico
Puerto Rico Department of Health
Secretary of Health
Phone No. (787) 274-7602
Fax No. (787) 250-6547

Rhode Island
Rhode Island Department of Health
Director of Health
Phone No. (401) 277-2231
Fax No. (401) 277-6548

South Carolina
SC Department of Health and Environmental Control
Commissioner
Phone No. (803) 734-4880
Fax No. (803) 734-4620

South Dakota
South Dakota State Dept of Health
Secretary of Health
Phone No. (605) 773-3361
Fax No. (605) 773-5683

Tennessee
Tennessee Department of Health
State Health Officer
Phone No. (615) 741-3111
Fax No. (615) 741-2491

Texas
Texas Department of Health
Commissioner of Health
Phone No. (512) 458-7375
Fax No. (512) 458-7477

Utah
Utah Dept of Health, Director
Phone No. (801) 538-6111
Fax No. (801) 538-6306

Vermont
Vermont Department of Health
Commissioner
Phone No. (802) 863-7280
Fax No. (802) 865-7754

Virgin Islands
Virgin Islands Department of Health
Commissioner of Health
Phone No. (340) 774-0117; Fax No. (340) 777-4001

Virginia
Virginia Department of Health
State Health Commissioner
Phone No. (804) 786-3561
Fax No. (804) 786-4616

K-26

Washington
Washington State Department of Health
Acting Secretary of Health
Phone No. (360) 753-5871
Fax No. (360) 586-7424

West Virginia
Bureau for Public Health
WV Department of Health & Human Resources
Commissioner of Health
Phone No. (304) 558-2971
Fax No. (304) 558-1035

Wisconsin
Division of Health
Wisconsin Department of Health and Family Services
Administrator
Phone No. (608) 266-1511
Fax No. (608) 267-2832

Wyoming
Wyoming Department of Health
Director
Phone No. (307) 777-7656
Fax No. (307) 777-7439

Order Form

Name: _____

Address: _____

City, State, Zip: _____

Daytime phone/email: _____

Personal Check or Credit Card (circle one):

               VISA   Mastercard   American   Express Discover

Card Number: _____

Expiration: _____ Signature:_____

TITLE	ISBN	PRICE	QUANTITY	SUBTOTAL
USAMRIID's Biological Casualties	1-58808-162-1	$ 9.95		
USAMRIID's Chemical Casualties	1-58808-168-0	$ 9.95		
AFRRI Radiological Casualties	1-58808-170-2	$ 9.95		
Healthy People 2010 – two volume set	1-883205-75-1 1-883205-78-6	$75.00		
U.S. Department of Health and Human Services Healthy People 2010 – paperback one combined volume	1-58808-110-9	$49.50		
Clinician's Handbook of Preventive Services, 2nd edition	1-883205-32-8	$20.00		
U.S. Public Health Service Guide to Clinical Preventive Services, 2nd edition	1-883205-13-1	$24.00		
United States Preventive Services Task Force				
			Subtotal	
Shipping and Handling $7.50 per 2010 hard cover set of two volumes				
Other titles: S&H $4.00 each				
			TOTAL	

Please include 5.75% sales tax for orders from the District of Columbia.

Send your order to: Reiter's Scientific & Professional Books
   2021 K Street, N.W., Washington, D.C. 20006

Information: 800-591-2713 Fax: 202-296-9103 E-mail: books@reiters.com

Order Form

Name: _____

Address: _____

City, State, Zip: _____

Daytime phone/email: _____

Personal Check or Credit Card (circle one):

VISA   Mastercard   American   Express Discover

Card Number: _____

Expiration: _____ Signature: _____

TITLE	ISBN	PRICE	QUANTITY	SUBTOTAL
USAMRIID's Biological Casualties	1-58808-162-1	$ 9.95		
USAMRIID's Chemical Casualties	1-58808-168-0	$ 9.95		
AFRRI Radiological Casualties	1-58808-170-2	$ 9.95		
Healthy People 2010 – two volume set	1-883205-75-1 1-883205-78-6	$75.00		
U.S. Department of Health and Human Services Healthy People 2010 – paperback one combined volume	1-58808-110-9	$49.50		
Clinician's Handbook of Preventive Services, 2nd edition	1-883205-32-8	$20.00		
U.S. Public Health Service Guide to Clinical Preventive Services, 2nd edition	1-883205-13-1	$24.00		
United States Preventive Services Task Force				
			Subtotal	
Shipping and Handling $7.50 per 2010 hard cover set of two volumes				
		Other titles: S&H $4.00 each		
			TOTAL	

Please include 5.75% sales tax for orders from the District of Columbia.

Send your order to: Reiter's Scientific & Professional Books
   2021 K Street, N.W., Washington, D.C. 20006

Information: 800-591-2713 Fax: 202-296-9103 E-mail: books@reiters.com

Order Form

Name: _____

Address: _____

City, State, Zip: _____

Daytime phone/email: _____

Personal Check or Credit Card (circle one):

      VISA   Mastercard   American   Express Discover

Card Number: _____

Expiration: _____ Signature: _____

TITLE	ISBN	PRICE	QUANTITY	SUBTOTAL
USAMRIID's Biological Casualties	1-58808-162-1	$ 9.95		
USAMRIID's Chemical Casualties	1-58808-168-0	$ 9.95		
AFRRI Radiological Casualties	1-58808-170-2	$ 9.95		
Healthy People 2010 – two volume set	1-883205-75-1 1-883205-78-6	$75.00		
U.S. Department of Health and Human Services Healthy People 2010 – paperback one combined volume	1-58808-110-9	$49.50		
Clinician's Handbook of Preventive Services, 2nd edition	1-883205-32-8	$20.00		
U.S. Public Health Service Guide to Clinical Preventive Services, 2nd edition	1-883205-13-1	$24.00		
United States Preventive Services Task Force				
			Subtotal	
Shipping and Handling $7.50 per 2010 hard cover set of two volumes				
Other titles: S&H $4.00 each				
			TOTAL	

Please include 5.75% sales tax for orders from the District of Columbia.

Send your order to: Reiter's Scientific & Professional Books
  2021 K Street, N.W., Washington, D.C. 20006

Information: 800-591-2713 Fax: 202-296-9103 E-mail: books@reiters.com